Lecture Notes in Biomathematics

ctd. on inside back cover

Lecture Notes in Biomathematics

Managing Editor: S. Levin

69

Steven H. Strogatz

The Mathematical Structure of the Human Sleep-Wake Cycle

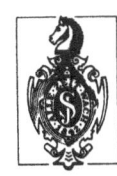

Springer-Verlag

Berlin Heidelberg New York London Paris Tokyo

Author

Steven H. Strogatz
Department of Mathematics
Harvard University
Cambridge, MA 02138, USA

ISBN-13:978-3-540-17176-8
DOI: 10.1007/978-3-642-46589-5

e-ISBN-13:978-3-642-46589-5

2146/3140-543210

ABSTRACT

The influence of the brain's circadian clock on sleep-wake timing has been clarified by experimental studies of subjects living for months in environments shielded from 24-hour time cues. The key finding is "internal desynchronization," in which the circadian rhythms of sleep and body temperature spontaneously adopt different periods. Although several theorists have claimed recently that their oscillator models account remarkably well for the sleep-wake data, disagreement persists about the experimental facts themselves, and about the standards of performance against which the models should be judged. This monograph addresses those two difficulties.

For the first time, much of the world literature on internal desynchronization is compiled and reanalyzed, revealing several patterns with implications for sleep research and circadian biology. The phase of the circadian pacemaker at bedtime determines the durations of sleep, prior wakefulness, and the wake-sleep cycle. The controversial relation of sleep length to prior wake length is clarified, thereby unifying results from synchronized and desynchronized subjects. Circadian phase-dependent rate functions for the sleep-wake transition are estimated, as are the frequency distributions for the timing of sleep onset and awakening. New methods for extracting circadian period and phase from sleep data alone are presented and validated. The most important empirical finding concerns a zone of the circadian cycle occurring 1-3h before habitual bedtime, in which subjects were virtually unable to fall asleep, suggesting that circadian phase dysfunction underlies certain insomnias.

We introduce the first analytically tractable model of sleep-wake timing, based on coupled nonlinear phase-only oscillators. Exact solutions are used to predict various empirical relationships. A second new model, based on beat phenomena, elucidates the influential and more complex models of Daan et al. and Kronauer et al. Phase plane and asymptotic analyses interconnect the models. Computer simulations indicate that the models of Kronauer et al. and Daan et al. perform no better than the two simple models, when tested against internal desynchronization data. However, a modification of the Daan model produces a superior fit to the desynchrony data. The analysis presented here establishes a rational framework for the evaluation of models of the human sleep-wake cycle.

Preface

Over the past three years I have grown accustomed to the puzzled look which appears on people's faces when they hear that I am a mathematician who studies sleep. They wonder, but are usually too polite to ask, what does mathematics have to do with sleep? Instead they ask the questions that fascinate us all: Why do we have to sleep? How much sleep do we really need? Why do we dream?

These questions usually spark a lively discussion leading to the exchange of anecdotes, last night's dreams, and other personal information. But they are questions about the *function* of sleep and, interesting as they are, I shall have little more to say about them here.

The questions that have concerned me deal instead with the *timing* of sleep. For those of us on a regular schedule, questions of timing may seem vacuous. We go to bed at night and get up in the morning, going through a cycle of sleeping and waking every 24 hours. Yet to a large extent, the cycle is imposed by the world around us. The question arises: What would we do if we could choose our own schedules, unconstrained by earthly periodicities? Would we still adhere to a 24 hour day? Or perhaps our sleeping and waking patterns would become random?

To answer such questions, "time-isolation" experiments have actually been performed, at first by having brave subjects live alone for weeks in underground caves or bunkers, without access to clocks or other information about the time of day, free to choose their own mealtimes and bedtimes. Nowadays the studies are conducted in specially designed, soundproofed, windowless apartments. While the approach may seem contrived, it has yielded important results with implications for the treatment of insomnia and the design of shift work schedules.

Time-isolation experiments are part of a long-term research strategy. The first goal is to understand the part played by our internal biological clocks in the control of the sleep-wake cycle; then we can aspire to consider the complexities of real life, where the sleep-wake cycle is also influenced by work schedules, light and darkness, alarm clocks, meals, social demands, ambient noise, sleeping pills, and so on.

Thus we restrict attention here to questions about the timing and duration of spontaneous sleep and wake, as manifested during time-isolation experiments. It is important to recognize that in addition to the exclusion of external schedulers, there are other simplifications inherent in this approach.

First, the events within sleep are ignored. Admittedly, a great deal of fascinating sleep research concerns the different stages of sleep: rapid eye-movement (REM) sleep, in which dreams occur; slow-wave sleep, the "deepest" stage which in pathological cases is associated with bedwetting, sleepwalking, and night terrors; and the lighter stages of non-REM sleep, which mediate the transitions between deep sleep, dreaming and wakefulness. However, the emphasis here is on sleep as distinct from wake, rather than on the internal organization of sleep itself.

Second, we shall not look inside the black box of the brain's biological machinery. Someday a complete theory of sleep will be formulated in terms of neurotransmitters, receptor kinetics, and so on. Indeed some of that story has already been worked out. But just as genetics and thermodynamics were successfully developed before the advent of molecular biology and statistical mechanics, the formal rules of sleep-wake timing may be discoverable even though their neurochemical basis is largely unknown.

It may seem implausible that any rules at all should underlie the timing of unrestricted sleep and wake. We all know that we can prolong wakefulness with a mere act of will. Indeed it may be that some of the unexplained scatter in the sleep-wake data reported here is due to such uncontrolled acts of volition. Yet within the scatter there is an astonishing amount of structure and pattern, much of which appears to be universal across subjects, and some of which is explicable in terms of simple mathematical oscillator models. It is the patterns lurking in the data, and their rationalization by oscillator theory, which shall concern us in the pages to follow. Along the way, we shall gain insights into the timing of sleep in our everyday lives — for example, why many of us feel sleepy in the mid-afternoon or why we often find it difficult to fall asleep on Sunday night.

Acknowledgments

I am grateful to the Division of Applied Sciences, Harvard University, for generous financial support.

For providing me with raw data from their experiments, it is with sincere appreciation that I thank Mary Carskadon; Scott Campbell; Peretz Lavie and Miriam Wollman; Ellie Hoey and the Cornell Institute of Chronobiology; and Chuck Czeisler.

Thank you to: Louise Kassabian and Maryorie Rosado, for four years of good humor and superb secretarial assistance; Joan Finkelstein, for digitizing several sleep-wake records; Margot Burrell and William Minty, for careful preparation of the figures; Armand Dionne, for photography with a smile; Renate D'Arcangelo, for painstaking preparation of the manuscript; Emery Brown, for talks, tennis, and statistical advice; Donald Anderson, for helpful criticism of a draft of this manuscript; Tom McMahon, for always coming to my rescue in matters academic; Chuck Czeisler, for laughter and for teaching me about circadian rhythms and scientific writing; Art Winfree, for being an inspiration and for innumerable lessons over the years; and my parents, for love and support.

I offer special thanks to Richard Kronauer, for discussions, assistance, encouragement, curiosity, and optimism. He had the seminal ideas for much of the work reported here, especially that in Chapters 3 and 4. In particular, he devised the cohort analysis (Section 4.4.2.2); discovered and named the wake-maintenance zones (Section 4.5); discovered the $\sim$ 20-day cycle in the sleep-wake record of Subject 3.2 (Figure 4-25); suggested the sleep onset clustering method of estimating the circadian period (Section 4.6); and elucidated the properties of split sleepers and nappers (Section 4.10).

Steven H. Strogatz
Cambridge, Massachusetts
June, 1986

Table of Contents

Chapter 1

Introduction

1.1 Beyond Time

In 1972, Michel Siffre spent six months alone in an underground cave. His account (Siffre, 1975) of that harrowing experience begins dramatically:

> Overcome with lethargy and bitterness, I sit on a rock and stare at my campsite in the bowels of Midnight Cave, near Del Rio, Texas. Behind me lie a hundred days of solitude; ahead loom two and a half more lonely months. But I — a wildly displaced Frenchman — know none of this, for I am living "beyond time," divorced from calendars and clocks, and from sun and moon, to help determine, among other things, the natural rhythms of human life.

One of these rhythms is the daily cycle of sleep and wake. In the constant conditions of his cave, Siffre was free of the 24h periodicities imposed by the outside world. Yet for 35 days, some *innate* rhythm kept Siffre on a regular "circadian" (= roughly daily) schedule. (Figure 1-1.) Notice however that it was not exactly 24h long. His sleep-wake timer ran slow, completing a cycle once every 26h or so. Then something odd happened on day 37. Siffre unknowingly skipped his usual bedtime, and stayed up for several extra hours. Then he slept and slept. (Strictly speaking, the data here reflect bedrest and activity, not sleep and wake — EEG brain wave data were recorded, but are not available.) This strange pattern of long wakes and sleeps occurred intermittently for the next month. Spontaneously, on day 63, he reverted to the steady 26h cycles. After nine more weeks, "wild variations" (Siffre, 1975) appeared again (day 130) and continued in "a seemingly random pattern" (Siffre, 1975) for 20 days. These again gave way (day 150) to a fairly regular 26h cycle, which persisted to the end of the experiment.

This record is absolutely remarkable. It raises many questions: why was Siffre's sleep-wake pattern sometimes regular, sometimes "random"? Are the random sections truly random, or subtly ordered? What physiological processes — in particular, what biological oscillators — kept Siffre on a 26h day, and what happened to them when "wild variations" broke out? To what extent can these patterns be explained mathematically?

1.2 The Rosetta Stone

The questions raised in the last section have intrigued physiologists, sleep researchers, and biomathematicians for the past 25 years. Many experiments like Siffre's have been performed in underground bunkers (Wever, 1979), caves (Mills *et al.*,1974; Jouvet *et al.*, 1974), and comfortable but soundproofed, windowless apartments (Webb and Agnew, 1974; Czeisler, 1978). In each case, the aim was to study human physiology, especially the sleep-wake cycle, in "free-running" conditions, with subjects shielded from periodic variations of the outside world and insulated from all knowledge of the time of day. The data which emerge are tantalizing — Winfree (1982b) has called them a "Rosetta Stone". Mathematicians entered the

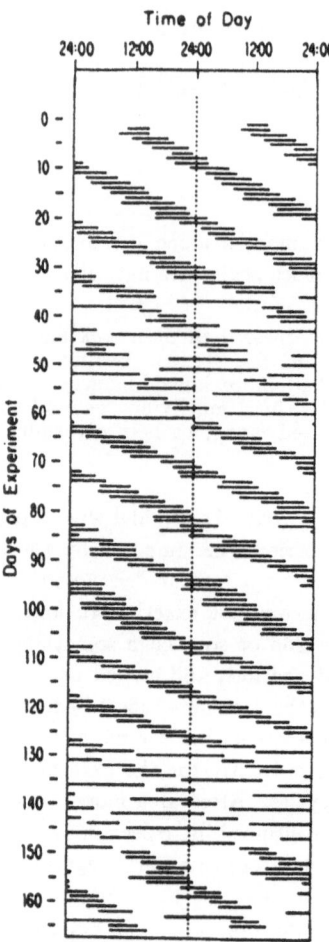

Figure 1-1. Sleep-wake record of Siffre's time-isolation study in Midnight Cave, Texas, 1972. Black bars represent times when Siffre was asleep. Each sleep episode is plotted twice: beneath the previous episode, and also to the right of it. This "double raster plot" emphasizes the continuity of the data across the artifactual edge at 24:00h.

Note that during the first 36 days, Siffre awoke later and later each day. Thus his sleep-wake cycle was longer than 24h, as indicated by the sloping of the black bars from upper left to lower right on the graph. (A vertical stacking of the bars would indicate a 24h period.)

On day 37, the sleep-wake pattern changed spontaneously. Subsequent chapters are devoted largely to an exploration of this phenomenon, known as "internal desynchronization."

For further information about the Siffre cave study, see Section 3.5.

fray in the 1980's, challenged by the riddles latent in the data of Czeisler (1978) and Wever (1979). The goal: to discover and explain the laws of human sleep-wake timing. In the subsequent outpouring of theory, many mathematical models were born. As will be seen, they tend to be abstract and phenomenological; theories at the neurochemical level must await a deeper understanding of the brain.

Recently the field hit an impasse — several modelers claimed that their formal black-box theories fit the facts remarkably well, yet consensus was limited by *two fundamental difficulties: few agreed about what the experimental facts were, and there were no shared standards for judging the success of a model's performance.*

1.3 Overview

The first half of this monograph is about experimental data drawn from studies of human subjects living in time-isolation. It attempts to remedy the lack of consensus about what phenomena need to be explained. The emphasis is on "spontaneous internal desynchronization," an amazing phenomenon in which the sleep-wake and temperature rhythms run with different periods, on average.

Chapter 2 provides background information: Its first section introduces terminology to be used throughout, and its second section summarizes the history of studies of free-running human sleep.

Chapter 3 is a data bank with annotations. I hope it will be useful to future researchers to have these data in one place. Many of the records, graphs and analyses have never been published before.

Chapter 4 distills the data of Chapter 3. I report several new regularities underlying the data and then review some previously proposed ones. The patterns reported here have implications for sleep research, circadian biology, and the treatment of insomnia. The chapter concludes with a list of the most salient, reliable facts about the free-running human sleep-wake cycle.

The second half of the monograph focuses on the issue of standards: how can one judge whether a model's verisimilitude is impressive, or only generic? By studying a variety of models, we can gain the perspective needed to assess the performance of particular ones.

Chapter 5 reviews previous models of the human circadian system, with special emphasis on the models of Kronauer *et al.* (1982, 1983) and Daan *et al.* (1984). Those two models continue to influence and even to polarize much of the current thinking about human sleep and circadian rhythms.

Chapter 6 uses graphical and asymptotic methods to analyze these two predominant models. In addition, two simpler alternatives are introduced to pinpoint the indispensable features of the more sophisticated models. The two simple models also act as "controls" when all four models are tested — they provide benchmarks which help us to evaluate the performance of the models of Kronauer *et al.* and Daan *et al.*.

Chapter 7 explores both new and old models with computer simulations, and compares their predictions to the empirical regularities established in Chapter 4. The main finding is that the models of Daan *et al.* (1984) and Kronauer *et al.* (1982, 1983) are scarcely more accurate than the simpler alternatives. All the models manage a qualitative fit to the data, but on more rigorous tests they all fail. Therefore quantitative predictions based on any of the models should be regarded skeptically. This cautionary note has practical implications because the models are being used by some researchers to guide the design of work schedules for pilots, policemen, and military personnel (Moore-Ede *et al.*, 1986).

Chapter 2

Experimental Background

2.1 Phenomena and Terminology

2.1.1 Introduction

To fix ideas and establish some standard jargon, this section consists of an annotated example. The notions introduced here recur throughout the rest of the text. Specialized terms are in italics; their meaning should be clear from context. For precise definitions, see Moore-Ede *et al.* (1982), Aschoff (1981), or Wever (1979) Glossary.

2.1.2 Example: A Six-month Record

Figure 2-1 shows the results of an experiment conducted by Czeisler, Weitzman, and Zimmerman at Montefiore Hospital, New York City (Kronauer *et al.*, 1983) in which a male human subject lived in a soundproofed, windowless, *time-isolation* facility for 6 months. For the first twenty days, the experimenters forced him to adhere strictly to his usual schedule. Each day he slept from 3:00 AM to 10:00 AM. Thus his *sleep-wake cycle* followed the usual 24h periodicity. Three meals and a snack were served each day. Lights were on during his waking hours, and off during bedrest. In other words, the illumination followed a 24h *light-dark cycle*.

Much of the subject's internal physiology varied with the time of day. For example, his *core body temperature*, measured continuously with a rectal thermometer, tended to rise during the day, and fall to minimum just before wake-up time. This *temperature rhythm* is remarkably stable and predictable. Of course, there are some day to day fluctuations in activity, exercise, etc., and these are reflected in the temperature — but such fluctuations really represent *evoked effects* on top of an underlying temperature oscillation. For example, sleep itself tends to lower body temperature, because of changes in posture and activity. But does this mean that with constant posture and inactivity the temperature rhythm would flatten and vanish?

The answer is no. This question was debated hotly (so to speak) for many years (reviewed in Czeisler, 1978; Aschoff, 1965); it is now recognized that core temperature does have an *endogenous* oscillatory component, as well as superimposed fluctuations evoked by showers, hot drinks, exercise, etc.

Returning to our example, on day 21 the subject was allowed to *free-run*: he could select his own bedtime, sleep for as long as he wanted, control the lights, and eat whenever hungry. He was thus shielded from the periodic signals — *zeitgebers* — that kept his bodily rhythms *entrained* to a 24h day. One constraint: he was told to avoid naps; sleeps were to be "for the night."

On this *self-selected* schedule, the subject tended to fall asleep later and later each day (a tendency familiar to many of us on the weekends). In this sense, the subject lost *external*

6

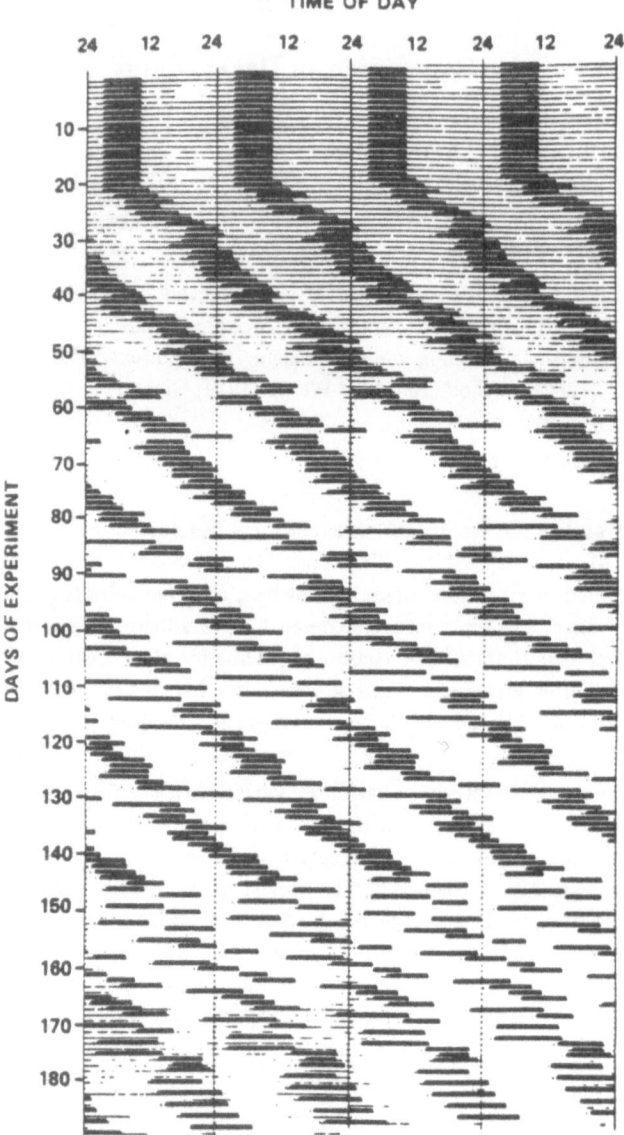

Figure 2-1. Sleep-wake record for subject LD03 (Section 3.2). Black bars represent sleep. Each sleep episode is plotted four times in a raster format. (See the legend to Figure 1-1 for an explanation of this method of presenting sleep-wake data.) Reproduced from Kronauer *et al.* (1983), Fig. 7, with permission.

synchronization to the outside world. The average *period* of his sleep-wake cycle was no longer 24h but about 25.3h. Halberg (1959) coined the term "circadian" for such roughly daily rhythms.

As for the subject's temperature rhythm, there was a change in *internal phase*: low temperature in free-run tended to occur near the *onset* of sleep, rather than just before wake-up (as observed in the first 20 days during 24h *entrainment*). This internal phase adjustment was achieved in the first few days after release from entrainment. Thereafter, temperature also adopted a 25.3h period, remaining *internally synchronized* to the sleep-wake cycle. During internal synchrony, rhythms of sleep and core body temperature have the same average period and a nearly constant *phase relationship*, i.e. sleep onset and low temperature are separated by a fixed time interval in each cycle.

If instead the phase relationship varies periodically, but the average periods remain equal, the subject is said to be *phase-trapped* (because the phase relation is trapped between the extremes of its cyclic variation). The subject in Figure 2-1 experienced intermittent phase-trapping on days 30–70.

Dramatic changes in the sleep-wake record occurred after day 82. The subject had *internally desynchronized*: the sleep-wake and temperature rhythms had different average periods, denoted τ_{SW} and τ_T, respectively. During clock days 82–92, $\tau_{SW} \simeq 30$h and $\tau_T \simeq 25.2$h. Thus the two rhythms drifted with respect to one another; though sleeps were often *phase-clustered* near low temperature, these clusters are punctuated by sleeps begun nearer to high temperature.

Note two points: **(1)** after desynchrony, τ_T shortened and τ_{SW} lengthened, relative to their values in synchrony. Because the common synchronized period lies between these, it is called the *compromise period*. **(2)** Sleep episodes initiated near low temperature were of typical ($\sim$ 7h) duration, while those begun at high temperature were extraordinarily long ($\sim$ 14h). In Chapter 4 much will be made of this relationship between sleep duration and *circadian phase* (the phase in the temperature cycle) at the time of sleep onset.

The subject's average sleep-wake period τ_{SW} continued to increase, until by the end of the record he was living on *bicircadian*, or roughly 48h cycles. Note the remarkably constant periodicity of those last 4 bicircadian cycles.

In contrast to the dramatic changes in the sleep-wake cycle, the temperature rhythm persisted stably throughout the entire free-run (Figure 2-2, unpublished figure kindly provided by C.A. Czeisler). Its average period, as determined by "minimum variance waveform eduction" (Czeisler, 1978) varied by about $\pm 1\%$ over six months! At first, during internal synchrony $\tau_T = 25.27$; from days 82–145, $\tau_T = 25.23$; and during days 145–189 when the subject was thoroughly desynchronized, $\tau_T = 25.03$.

The main observation to be made is that τ_T shortened as τ_{SW} increased, a trend observed to hold quite generally (Section 4.9.1). One interpretation is that during desynchrony τ_T is less influenced by evoked effects of the slower sleep-wake cycle. In this view, τ_T during desynchrony more nearly reflects the *intrinsic period* of the endogenous pacemaker driving the temperature rhythm.

TIME OF DAY

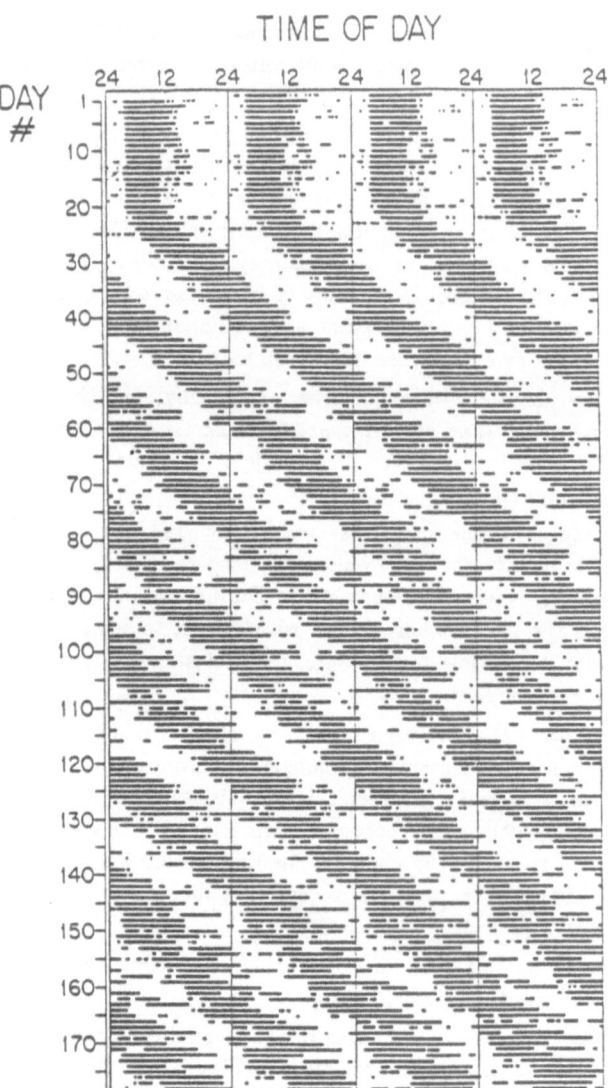

Figure 2-2. Low-temperature record for subject LD03 (Section 3.2). Black bars represent times when the subject's body temperature fell below the mean established in the first 20 days of the experiment (when subject was constrained to his usual 24h cycle with a 7h sleep episode each day, beginning at 3 AM; for full sleep-wake record, see Figure 2-1).

2.2 History of Free-Run Studies

This brief section sketches the history of major experimental studies of man's circadian timing system. The picture is drawn with broad strokes; for detailed review, see Czeisler (1978), Moore-Ede *et al.* (1982), Aschoff (1965), or Wever (1979). Though the history is recounted only briefly here, the *results* of all relevant studies will be examined in detail in Chapters 3 and 4.

2.2.1 Circadian Biology, 1950-1960

The 1950's witnessed intense activity and exciting discoveries in circadian biology. The state of the field at that time is well documented by the papers given at the Cold Spring Harbor Symposium on Biological Clocks (Volume **25**, 1960). At every turn, circadian rhythms were being found in plants and animals, and their properties were catalogued and compared. Experimenters subjected organisms to constant conditions of total darkness or never-ending light; perturbed them with blasts of light, chemicals, or temperature in order to phase-shift rhythms and examine their stability; and probed their limits of entrainment to various light-dark cycles and other zeitgebers. One question that was studied vigorously concerns the possible exogenous vs. endogenous source of circadian rhythms. It is universally agreed today that circadian rhythms are generated within the organism, and not by some subtle influence of the spin of the earth or other geophysical factors. The decisive arguments were provided by the extensive data showing a genetic basis for circadian rhythmicity, and by studies documenting the uniqueness of free-running period for each species and each individual within the species (reviewed by Moore-Ede *et al.*, 1982).

2.2.2 First Studies of Human Circadian Rhythms

In the early 1960's, two groups began to investigate the possibility that man, like other animals, possesses a circadian clock. The groups of Aschoff in Germany and Siffre in France both realized the importance of separating subjects from all possible factors which could act as zeitgebers. It is not easy to shut out the world so completely; Siffre (1964) himself lived in an underground cavern for two months in the summer of 1962, and Aschoff and Wever (1962) placed subjects in a soundproofed, sealed chamber in the basement of a Munich hospital. Temperature, urinary electrolytes, and activity-rest cycles (as opposed to polygraphically verified sleep-wake cycles) were recorded in these early studies, and revealed that man does have circadian rhythms and that his free-running "day" tends to exceed 24h.

Aschoff (1965) reported the next major discovery, a true breakthrough: spontaneous internal desynchronization. The implications were shocking: the internal phase map (Halberg, 1960) of desynchronized individuals might be completely disrupted, with physiologic rhythms peaking at inappropriate times with respect to one another. The untoward consequences — if any — to the individual remain conjectural (Kripke, 1983). There is even some indication of a "paradoxical" improvement in mood and performance during desynchronization (Wever, 1982a).

Aschoff (1965) found that his desynchronized subject's internal temporal order was not altogether lost — rhythms of temperature, urinary potassium and water excretion all free-ran at the same circadian period of 24.7h, while calcium excretion and activity showed a much slower rhythm, in excess of 32h. Similar results were obtained in many other experiments (Wever, 1979), leading to today's conventional view that man's circadian timing system is dominated by two oscillators (Moore-Ede et al., 1982).

Meanwhile Siffre's group was continuing its series of cave studies (Siffre et al., 1966). Their subjects endured several months of isolation, far longer than the one month indoor studies of Aschoff and coworkers, and lived amidst frigid temperatures, high humidity, and bat guano (Siffre, 1964; 1975). Himself the subject of the elaborate six-month, NASA-assisted study in Midnight Cave, Texas, Siffre (1975) wrote that he suffered from severe lapses of memory, weakened eyesight, a chronic squint, and psychological wounds, even months after the study was completed.

The full results of these cave studies have not been published in detail by the French group. In what has been published, they have documented several instances of internal desynchronization, and its complex evolution over several months. Siffre's (1975) 6-month record (Figure 1-1 and Section 3.5) is especially remarkable, because it shows two distinct desynchronies separated by several weeks of spontaneous re-synchronization. In the 4-month record of subject JC (Jouvet et al., 1974), the French group documented the marvelous, gradual unfolding of a sleep-wake cycle whose period increased monotonically, until a nearly bicircadian day was achieved (cf. Section 3.4).

2.2.3 Later Studies of Czeisler and Weitzman

In work at Montefiore Hospital, New York City in the 1970's and later at the Institute of Chronobiology, Cornell Medical Center, White Plains, New York and at the Harvard Medical School, Weitzman, Czeisler, and colleagues refined and extended all previous studies of human circadian rhythms.

Like Aschoff and Wever, they used a specially designed, fully equipped laboratory as the time-isolation environment; like Siffre et al., they traced the evolution of desynchrony for up to six months; like Webb and Agnew (1974), they measured the EEG of free-running subjects. But Czeisler and Weitzman went beyond earlier work — they polygraphically recorded sleep and sleep stages during internal desynchronization and correlated the internal organization of sleep with the timing of other simultaneously measured physiologic and neuroendocrine functions. In this way they investigated circadian influences on sleep regulation, for example, the close links between the circadian temperature rhythm, the duration of sleep, and REM propensity (Czeisler et al., 1980a). These results extended earlier reports (Wever, 1979) of an ongoing, residual modulation of sleep by the circadian temperature pacemaker, even during desynchrony when the two rhythms had ostensibly "uncoupled." Czeisler and Weitzman later applied the circadian principles gleaned from these studies to industrial medicine (Czeisler et al., 1982) and the treatment of certain sleep-onset insomnias (Czeisler et al., 1981).

Chapter 3
Data Bank

Format of the Data Bank

This chapter contains both raw data and analyses of many sleep-wake records. The emphasis is on internally desynchronized subjects, with a few examples of nappers and split sleepers. The subjects are discussed one at a time, whereas in the next chapter their records are pooled and general patterns are extracted.

For each subject, the analysis is divided into Remarks, Statistics and Graphs.

A. Remarks

Some subjects are of special historical or theoretical interest. A few remarks are offered, explaining why the subject is important, and mentioning any relevant information about experimental protocol, special problems posed by the data, etc.

B. Statistics

A summary of some important numbers characterizing the subject and the experimental record. Unavailable information is denoted by "N/A".

$N =$ number of sleep-wake cycles used in the analysis. Often only internally desynchronized sections of the record are considered. When synchronized, mildly desynchronized, or almost bicircadian sections co-exist in a record, the notations "synch", "de", or "bi" are used to distinguish them.

$\bar{\rho}, \bar{\alpha} =$ mean length of observed sleep and wake episodes. In nearly all cases, "sleep" and "wake" are more properly called "rest" and "activity" — even when EEG recordings were taken, they usually were unavailable for analysis.

$F =$ average sleep fraction $= \bar{\rho}/(\bar{\alpha} + \bar{\rho})$. Most of the time this number is close to 1/3, since subjects sleep about a third of the time.

$\tau_{SW} =$ average sleep-wake cycle period $= \bar{\alpha} + \bar{\rho}$. The standard deviation of the period (as measured from bedtime to bedtime) is also reported.

$\tau =$ average period of the circadian pacemaker during desynchrony. A period indicated by "minimum variance waveform eduction of temperature" (Czeisler, 1978) is the standard estimate of τ, but there are other estimates based on sleep data alone (Section 4.6) which supplement the temperature estimate. They become especially important when temperature data are scant (minima only) or lacking altogether. The estimates derived from sleep data are based on (1) the period which yields the maximum phase-clustering of sleep onsets and (2) the period which yields the tightest relation between sleep length and circadian phase. These methods are explained in detail in Section 4.6.

Sex/Age: Note that most of the subjects are males in their 20's.

Code: The initials or designation of the subject. Often the same subjects are discussed in different publications — a knowledge of their code names allows one to keep track of them (see e.g. PR01, Section 3.1).

Source: Original reference from which the record was obtained. Sometimes several are listed — these offer further analysis or information. No attempt has been made to be comprehensive, though most of the key references are listed.

C. Graphs

For each subject, a few sorts of graphs are presented, each helpful in analyzing some aspect of the sleep-wake record. **Note:** In general, only internally desynchronized sections of the records are considered.

24 Hour Raster Plots

The familiar 24h "raster plot" or "actogram" shows when rest and activity occurred on each day (Figure 3-1). Other information such as the timing of the circadian temperature minimum can be shown conveniently on the same graph. For many of the subjects, such raster plots are available in the published literature, and are not repeated here. Only unpublished or unusually long (Figure 3-1) records are presented in 24h raster format. Instead, our standard representation for all human free-run data is a "normalized raster."

Normalized Raster

One problem with the usual raster plot is its dependence on a periodicity (24h) which is physiologically irrelevant during free-run. The important timescale is the period of the circadian temperature cycle. For example, sleep often begins near the temperature trough. Because the temperature rhythm typically has a period near 25h, sleep and temperature appear to slope diagonally down the raster (Figure 3-2). This diagonal sloping is inconvenient. The eye does not compare points on the same diagonal line as easily as those on the same vertical line. Moreover, subtle changes in period and phase are hard to spot in the usual representation.

Therefore the free-run data have been replotted on a circadian basis (Figure 3-2). The sleep-wake cycle is plotted on a raster with a repeat interval equal to the period of the circadian temperature cycle. Thus all points on the same vertical line correspond to the same circadian phase. Next the arbitrary zero of the time variable is chosen to align the mid-trough of the averaged temperature cycle with the vertical midline of the raster plot.

With these normalizations, it becomes easy to compare records of internal desynchronization which had appeared dissimilar (Figure 3-3). Temperature troughs suddenly line up; long sleeps can be seen to occur near high temperature; short sleeps begin near low temperature; and there are two invariant zones where these subjects never fall asleep. In other words, both the length of a sleep episode and the time of retiring are influenced strongly by the circadian pacemaker, marked by the circadian temperature cycle. These points will be elaborated in Chapter 4. For now, they motivate the introduction of another type of graph

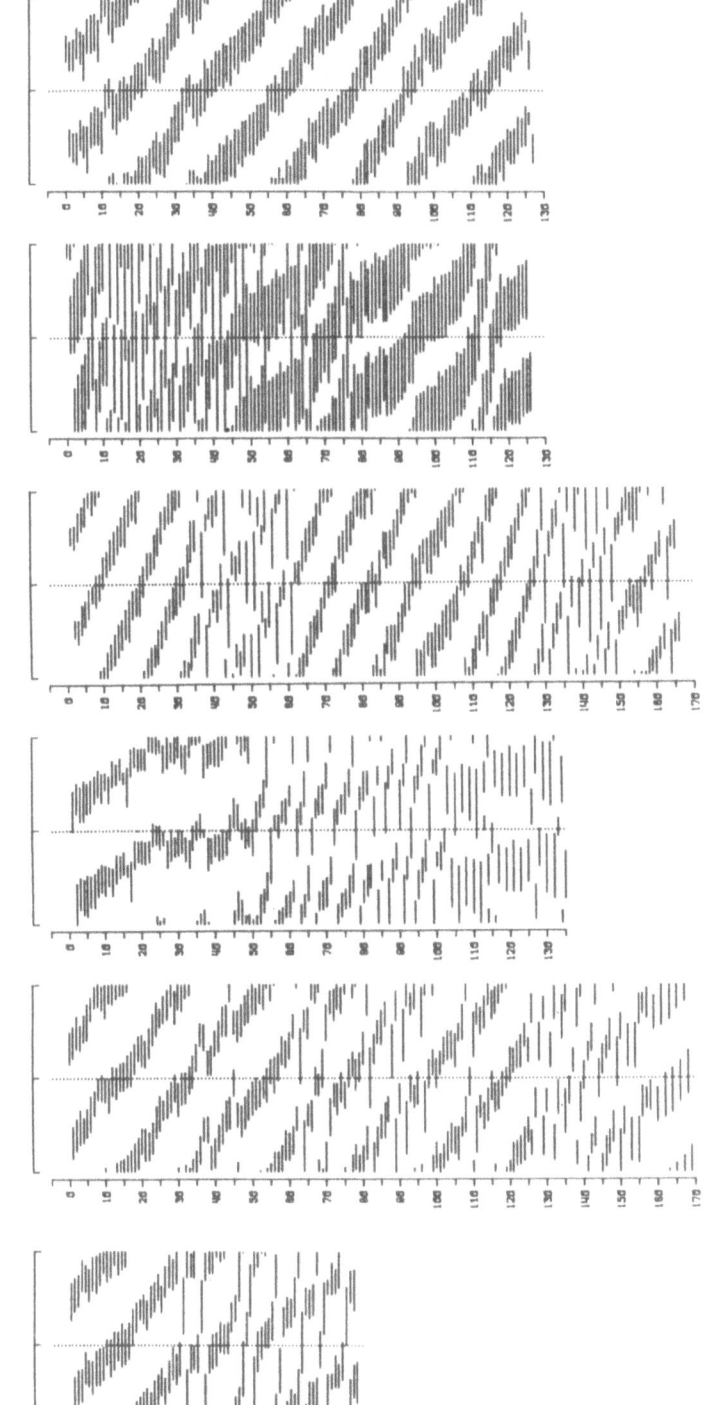

Figure 3-1. Sleep-wake raster plots for Subjects 3.1, 3.2, 3.4, 3.5, 3.16, and 3.17, respectively. See Figure 1-1 for explanation of 24h raster format.

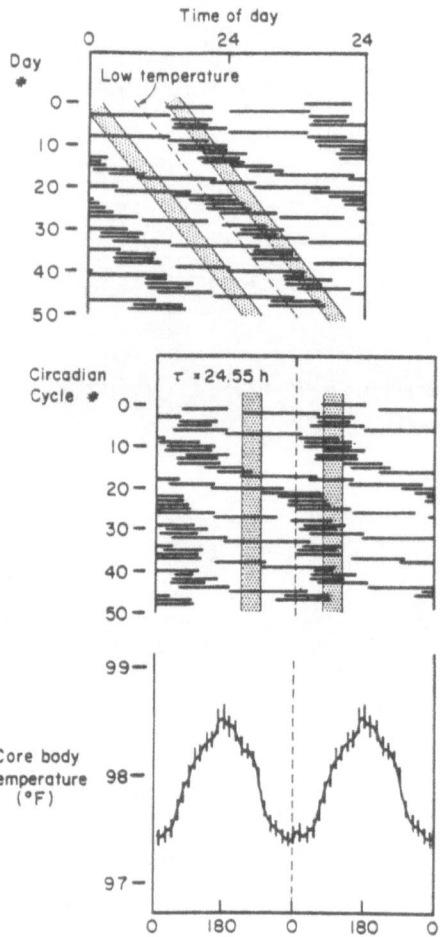

Figure 3-2. (top): A conventional 24h raster plot of a sleep-wake record. Data are shown for PR01 (Section 3.1) during internal desynchronization. Black bars represent sleep. Successive days are plotted beneath one another, and the entire record is offset and double-plotted to the right. The dashed line locates the mid-trough of the educed temperature rhythm. Parallel to it are stippled bands, phases in the circadian temperature cycle at which sleep never begins.

(middle): Normalized raster plot of the same record. The record is replotted at a repeat of 24.55h, the average period of the temperature cycle. The mid-trough of the average temperature rhythm is located by the dashed vertical line at the center of the figure.

(bottom): The educed (average) temperature rhythm (mean ± S.E.), plotted in a cycle of 360 degrees. In subsequent figures we usually divide the circadian cycle into 25 circadian hours instead of 360 degrees. Mid-low temperature occurs at phase 0.

15

Phase of circadian cycle

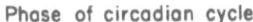

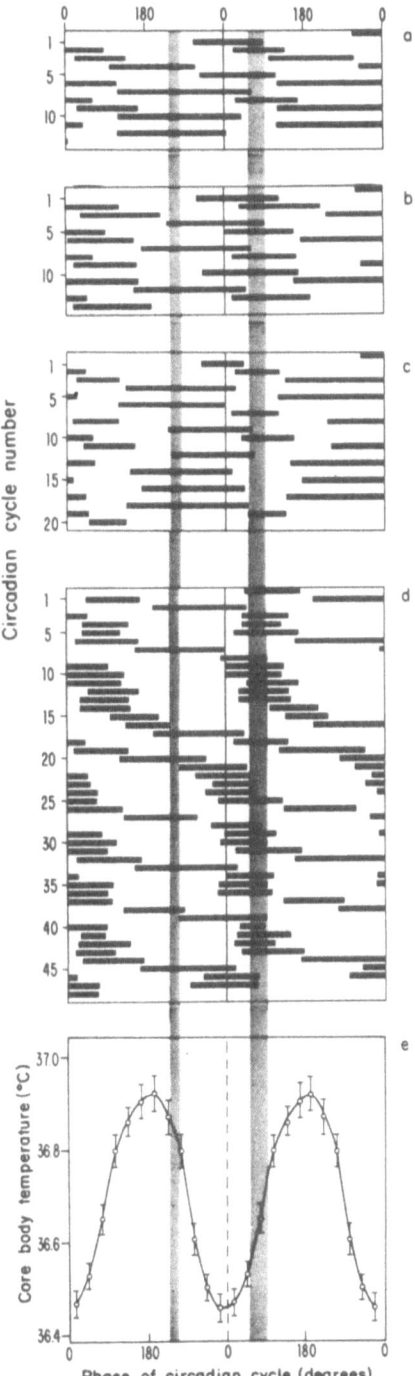

Figure 3-3. (a–d) Normalized raster plots of sleep-wake records from internally desynchronized subjects. Stippled vertical bands show zones of the circadian cycle where sleep onset is virtually forbidden (see Section 4.5).

(e) Average waveform of body temperature for the desynchronized subjects of (a–d).

For details about the subjects, see Legend to Figure 4-11.

which will be presented for each desynchronized subject.

Sleep Length and Circadian Phase

To quantify the dependence of sleep length (ρ) on the circadian phase of sleep onset (ϕ_s), the circadian cycle has been divided into 25 "circadian hours," with phase $\phi = 0 = 25$ at the mid-trough of the temperature rhythm. Then the length of each sleep episode is plotted as a function of the circadian phase at which it begins (e.g., Section 3.1, Figure 3-5). Where possible the $\phi_s{:}\rho$ graph is aligned vertically with the corresponding normalized raster for easy comparison.

The $\phi_s{:}\rho$ graph also allows a rapid inspection of the relation between bedtime preference and circadian phase. For example, the dense cluster of points near $\phi = 0$ in Figure 3-5 indicates at a glance the high sleep propensity near low temperature. For more precise ways to quantify sleep propensity, see Sections 4.4, 4.5, and 4.6.

Organization of Data Bank

The first 15 subjects form the *core* of the data bank (Table 3-1). All of them exhibited spontaneous internal desynchronization with a long sleep-wake cycle. Their records provide the raw data from which the empirical patterns of Chapter 4 are extracted. Subjects 16 and 17 are long (4 months) records of free-run, but they are not included among the core subjects. In one case the reported data are dubious and in the other internal desynchronization never occurred. Subjects 18–22 showed napping or split sleep patterns, a qualitatively different behavior from the core subjects. These subjects with short sleep-wake cycle are analyzed collectively in Section 4.10.

Sources of Data

C.A. Czeisler and colleagues of the late E.D. Weitzman kindly provided the raw data for Subjects 1–3, 7–9, and 17–20. Bedrest data for Subject 16 were provided by A.T. Winfree, who obtained the original records from D.S. Minors. Data for all other subjects were obtained by laborious digitizing of enlarged photographic reproductions of the published records. It should be recognized that such a procedure is susceptible to a number of systematic errors; therefore greater confidence should be assigned to those analyses below which are based on the data of Czeisler and Weitzman.

Table 3-1: Spontaneous internal desynchronization with lengthening of activity/rest cycle.

Subject	Code	N	$\bar{\rho}$	$\bar{\alpha}$	F	τ_{SW}	τ
1	PR01	40	9.1	20.3	0.31	29.4±5.2	24.5
2(de)	LD03	52	7.9	20.5	0.28	28.3±5.5	25.2
2(bi)	LD03	31	8.2	26.7	0.23	34.9±8.9	25.0
3	426F	18	12.2	23.6	0.34	35.8±4.8	24.7
4(de)	JC	38	7.7	23.0	0.25	30.6±5.0	24.3
4(bi)	JC	19	11.2	30.3	0.27	41.5±9.9	24.3
5(de1)	MS	21	9.8	23.2	0.30	33.0±8.6	25.6
5(de2)	MS	16	10.4	25.0	0.29	35.5±6.1	25.3
6	KD	17	9.9	19.3	0.34	29.1±4.8	25.2
7	FR03	8	13.9	24.2	0.36	38.1±7.3	25.1
8	FR04	9	13.4	23.6	0.36	37.0±4.0	24.3
9	FR10	12	11.8	28.0	0.30	39.8±6.5	24.3
10	N/A	17	10.7	21.7	0.33	32.4±5.6	24.5
11	N/A	11	11.7	20.0	0.37	31.8±4.6	24.9
12	EvS	15	9.2	24.0	0.28	33.1±4.2	25.1
13	F	16	12.3	20.8	0.37	33.1±5.1	24.7
14	G6	8	11.7	23.1	0.34	34.8±6.3	25.1
15	HN	7	14.0	21.9	0.39	35.9±5.4	24.9

Total: 355

3.1 Subject 1 (PR01)

Remarks

This record has influenced much of the theorizing of Kronauer *et al.* (1982, 1983) about internal desynchronization. Many phenomena are displayed in a gradual, almost stately procession: synchrony with internal phase drift gives way to apparent phase-trapping, followed by internal desynchrony with an unusually clear pattern of "beats." Kronauer *et al.* have made at least three different simulations of this record (cf. Section 5.3).

The record of PR01 has been published so often to the exclusion of others that one might imagine it to be the typical example of free-run. In fact this record is special in many ways, as should be clear from an examination of the other records in this chapter.

Statistics

	N	$\bar{\rho}$	$\bar{\alpha}$	F	τ_{SW}
phase-trapping/synch	28	8.2	17.0	0.32	25.2±2.2
desynch	40	9.1	20.3	0.31	29.4±5.2

τ estimate: 24.55

temp.(eduction)	sleep onsets	sleep length
24.55	24.40	24.55

Sex	Age	Code	Source
M	23	PR01	Czeisler, 1978 — Fig. 19
			Czeisler *et al.*, 1980a — Fig. 1
			Kronauer *et al.*, 1982 — Fig. 1A
			Moore-Ede *et al.*, 1982 — Fig. 6.4A
			Kronauer *et al.*, 1983 — Fig. 1
			Kronauer, 1984 — Fig. 4A
			Strogatz *et al.*, 1986 — Fig. 1

OFFSET INTERVAL = 24.00 HRS

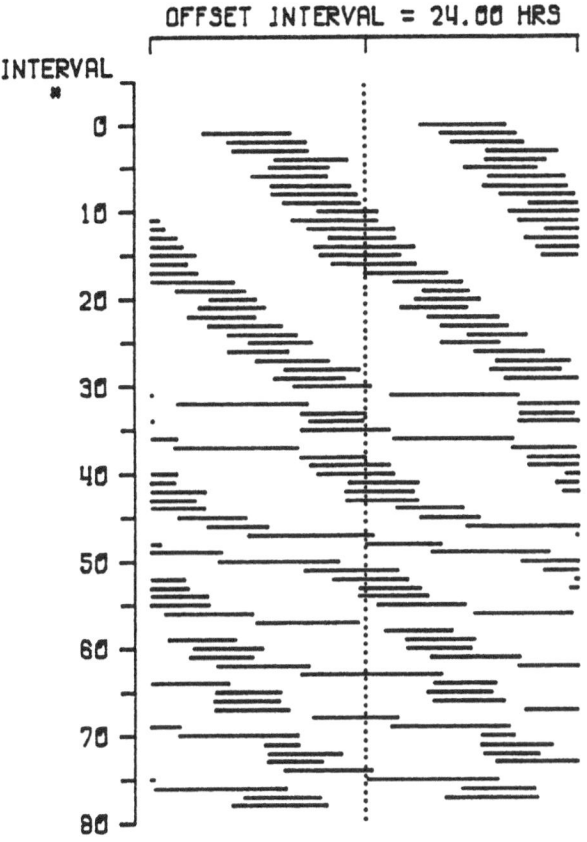

Figure 3-4. 24h raster plot for Subject 3.1.

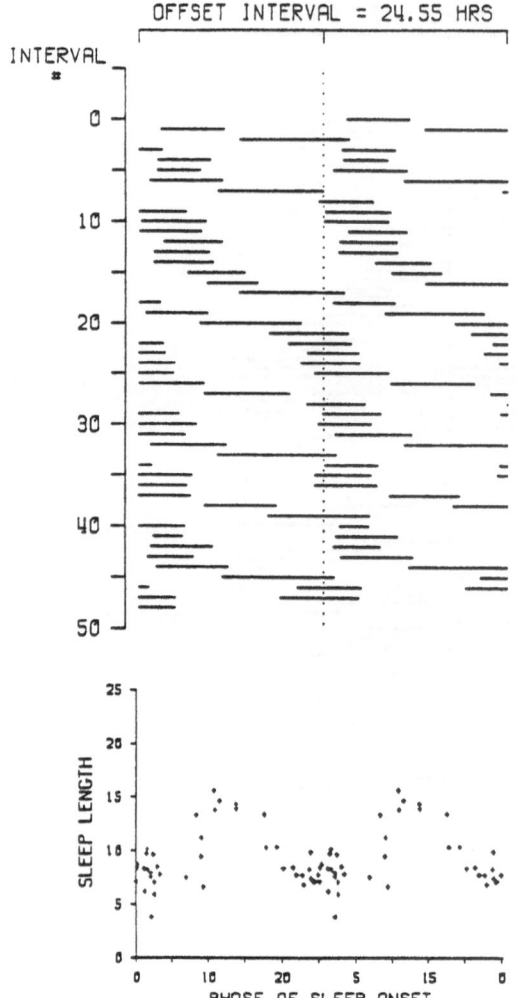

Figure 3-5. (top): Normalized raster for Subject 3.1. Only the last 40 sleep-wake cycles, when the subject was internally desynchronized, are shown here. For explanation of normalization, see Figure 3-2 .

(bottom): The length of each sleep episode is plotted as a function of the phase in the circadian cycle at bedtime. Note that short sleeps begin near low temperature (phase = 0), and long sleeps begin near high temperature.

3.2 Subject 2 (LD03)

Remarks

This six-month record is magnificent. I have divided it into three sections according to the sleep-wake behavior: synchrony/phase-trapping; mild desynchrony; and strong desynchrony/bicircadian (cf. Subject 3.4). The many phenomena displayed here have already been discussed in Section 2.1.2.

Despite dramatic fluctuations in the timing of activity across the three sections of the record, the period of the temperature cycle (25.1 ± 0.1) varied by less than 1%!

Note the stunning bicircadian synchronization in the final 5 cycles. No other subject is as regular in this respect. The sleep fraction dropped to a tiny 0.21 in this section.

The average sleep-wake cycle period tended to increase over the course of the experiment, but appears to have been modulated by a ~ 20 day cycle (cf. Figure 4-25).

The dot at cycle #8 of the strong desynchrony section signifies that the subject was caught napping without EEG hook-up for an unknown duration. Note that the "nap" actually occurred near the temperature trough.

In the ϕ_s:ρ plot of Figure 3-7, the crosses mark data from the mildly desynchronized section of record (Figure 3-7, top left), and the triangles mark data from the strong desynchrony (Figure 3-7, top right).

Statistics

	N	$\bar{\rho}$	$\bar{\alpha}$	F	τ_{SW}
phase-trapping	28	7.3	18.0	0.29	25.3±2.9
mild desynch	52	7.9	20.5	0.28	28.3±5.5
strong desynch	31	8.2	26.7	0.23	34.9±8.9
last 5 cycles of strong desynch	5	10.5	39.5	0.21	50.5±0.7

τ estimate: 25.03

temp.(education)	sleep onsets	sleep length
25.27 (phase-trapping)	25.25	25.30
25.23 (mild desynch)	25.15	25.2
25.03 (strong desynch)	24.85 major peak	24.9
	25.05 minor peak	

Sex	Age	Code	Source
M	24	LD03	Kronauer *et al.*, 1983 — Fig. 7
			Kronauer, 1984 — Fig. 2

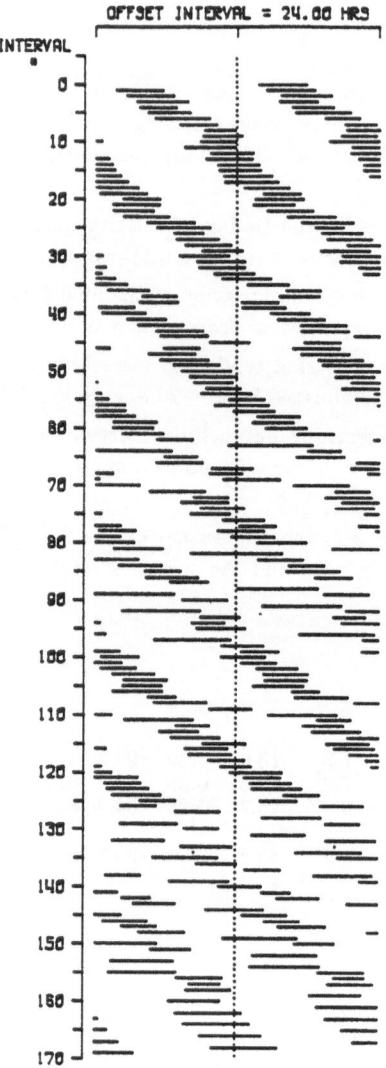

Figure 3-6. 24h raster plot for Subject 3.2.

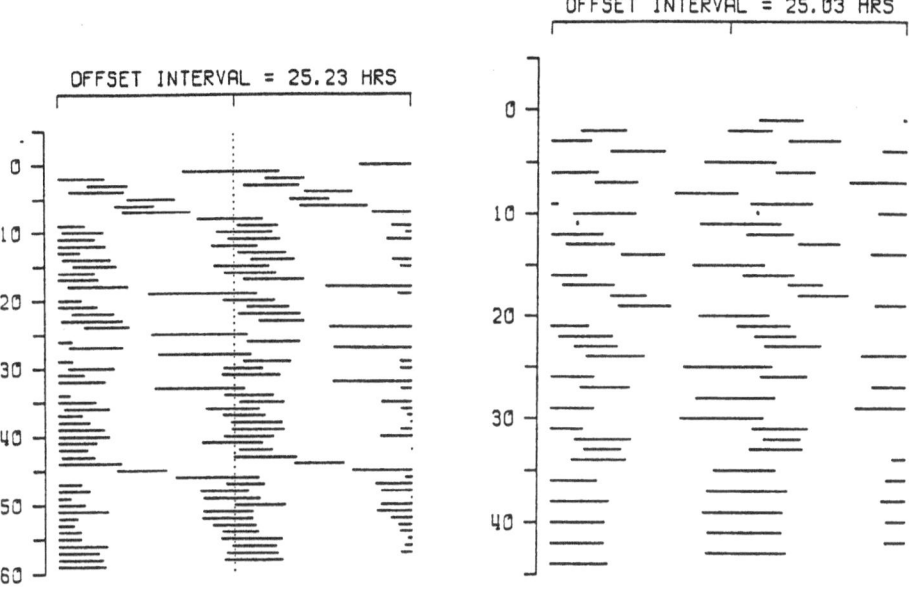

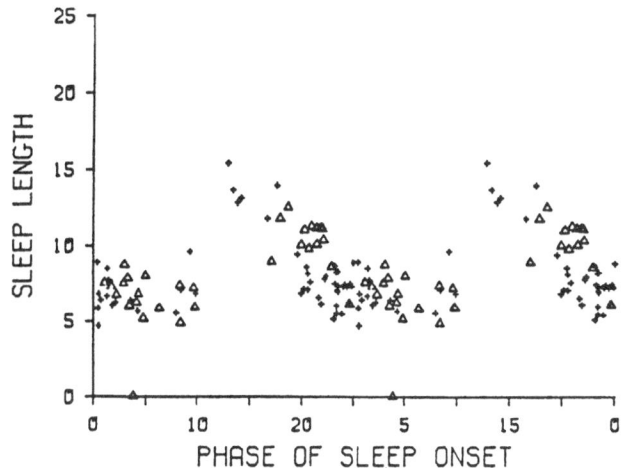

Figure 3-7. Normalized rasters and sleep duration data for Subject 3.2.

3.3. Subject 3 (426F)

Remarks

This recent experiment validates the "constant routine" method of assessing circadian phase by comparing it to results obtained from temperature waveform eduction during desynchrony.

Constant routines (Czeisler *et al.*, 1985, 1986) were performed on three occasions. The first two "endogenous circadian phase assessments" (CR1 and CR2, Figure 3-8) took place during 24h-entrainment in the laboratory. The temperature minimum occurred later on the second measurement than the first. One possible explanation is that the laboratory zeit-gebers are weaker than those of the outside world, and hence the circadian cycle drifted later (almost free-running) in response to the weaker coupling to the environment. This internal phase adjustment during laboratory entrainment has been observed on other occasions (Czeisler *et al.*, 1986).

On the last constant routine (CR3), two temperature minima were recorded. A thin dashed line was extrapolated between these minima and that obtained on the second constant routine, yielding an average period of 24.60h for the temperature cycle. The phase and period from this two point measurement agreed nicely with the values obtained from temperature eduction (large dashes, Figure 3-8) over the entire record.

Statistics

	N	$\bar{\rho}$	$\bar{\alpha}$	F	τ_{SW}
desynch	18	12.2	23.6	0.34	35.8±4.8

τ estimate: 24.68

temperature	sleep onsets	sleep length
24.68 (eduction)	24.80	24.90
24.60 (constant routines)		

Sex	Age	Code	Source
M	23	426F	Czeisler *et al.*, 1986

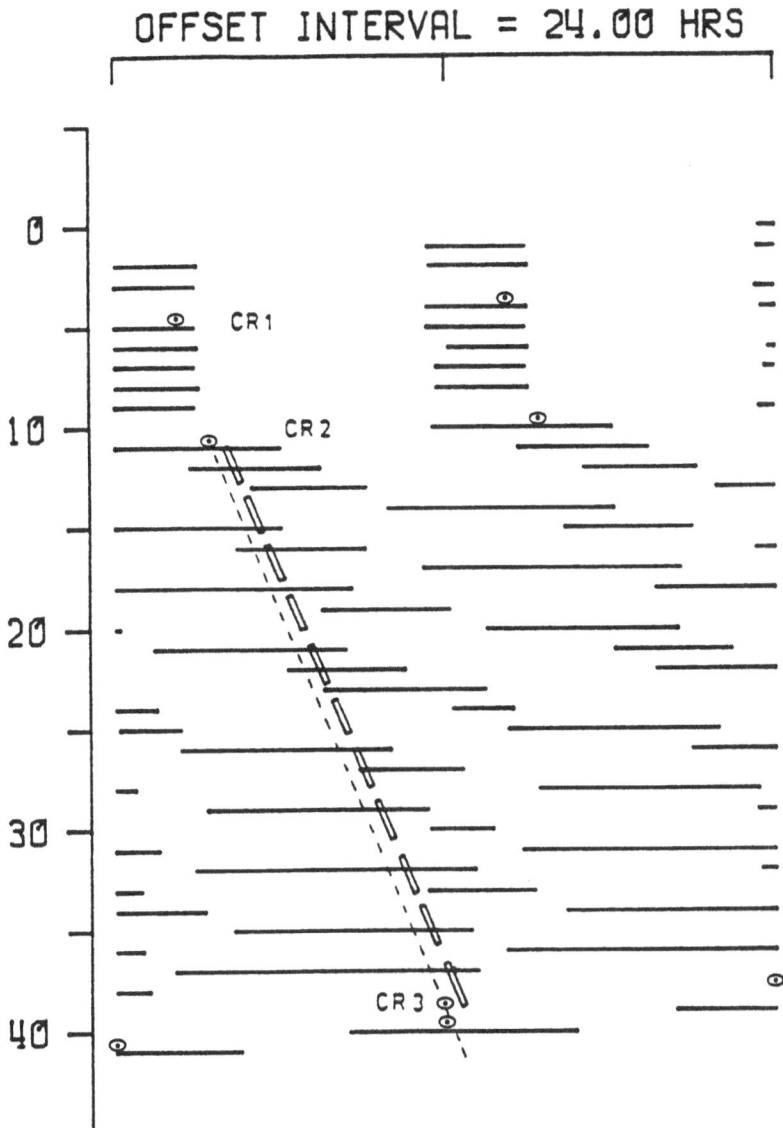

Figure 3-8. 24h raster for Subject 3.3. Encircled dots, temperature minima estimated during constant routine (Czeisler *et al.*, 1986).

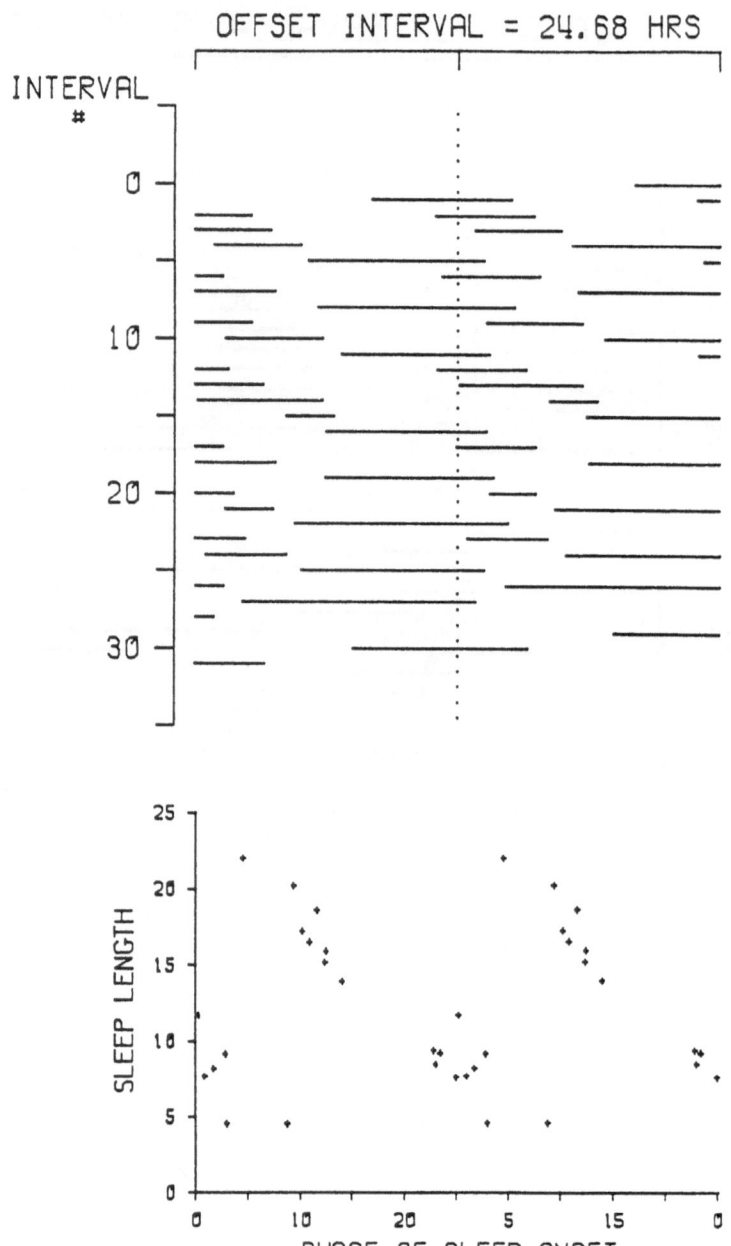

Figure 3-9. Normalized raster and sleep duration data for Subject 3.3.

3.4 Subject 4 (Jouvet JC)

Remarks

JC was a subject in a cave study led by Michel Siffre. The object of the study was to gain more information about the "bicircadian rhythm" which another subject, J.P. Mairetet, had adopted spontaneously during an earlier pilot cave study. Those initial results struck the French researchers as very exciting, since they suggested that man could live on a 48h day but perceive it to be no longer than normal.

Subject JC seems to have been something of a disappointment to the investigators. Because he did not spontaneously reach a bicircadian rhythm after 33 cycles, the experimenters tried to provoke him into it by turning on the lights (500 watt bulb) around the clock until the end of the experiment.

Ironically, JC has turned out to be one of the most revealing subjects in the whole literature of human free-run studies. Like LD03 (Section 3.2), he showed a little of everything: synchrony, phase-trapping, desynchrony, and bicircadian cycles. Moreover, the stages unfolded in an orderly and tantalizing progression, as emphasized by Czeisler's (1978) beautiful figure in which 8 different sleep-wake records assemble to complete the jigsaw puzzle which is JC (see Figure 4-23).

No temperature data are available for JC. In another coup, Czeisler (1978) found a way to extract the presumed circadian periodicity of the temperature cycle from the sleep data alone (see Section 4.6). Winfree (1982c; 1984) has illustrated Czeisler's idea with dramatic graphics of his own.

One nice theoretical point illustrated by JC: the relation between sleep length and phase (Figure 3–11) is invariant throughout the record even though the outward appearance of the record metamorphoses steadily. This suggested to Winfree (1983) that the slow changes in sleep-wake behavior "may lie exclusively in the mechanism determining sleep onset (the duration of waking)." In Figure 3-11, crosses denote data from the desynchronized section of the record (circadian cycles 53-102), and triangles denote data from the bicircadian section (circadian cycles 102- end).

Other Tidbits: The cave that JC lived in was 65 m underground, and was frigid (6 ° C) and damp (100% relative humidity). He kept a fascinating diary, excerpted in Siffre (1972), in which he philosophizes about the meaning of free-run (obey physiology slavishly vs. exert some free will to override it) and tells about being awakened in the middle of the night by a telephone call from the experimenters, who instructed him to remove his EEG electrodes because an electrical storm was approaching.

Statistics

	N	$\bar{\rho}$	$\bar{\alpha}$	F	τ_{SW}
synch	17	7.3	17.5	0.29	24.9±3.2
phase-trapping	35	6.0	18.4	0.25	24.4±2.9
desynch	38	7.7	23.0	0.25	30.6±5.0
bicircadian	19	11.2	30.3	0.27	41.5±9.9

τ estimate: 24.27

temperature	sleep onsets	sleep length
N/A	24.4	24.27

Sex	Age	Code	Source
M	23	JC	Jouvet et al., 1974 — Fig. 2
			Chouvet et al., 1974
			Siffre, 1972 — Fig. 36
			Czeisler, 1978 — Fig. 23, 81
			Kronauer et al., 1982 — Fig. 1B
			Winfree, 1982a — Fig. 1
			Winfree, 1983 — Fig. 5
			Moore-Ede et al., 1982 — Fig. 6.4B

OFFSET INTERVAL = 24.00 HRS

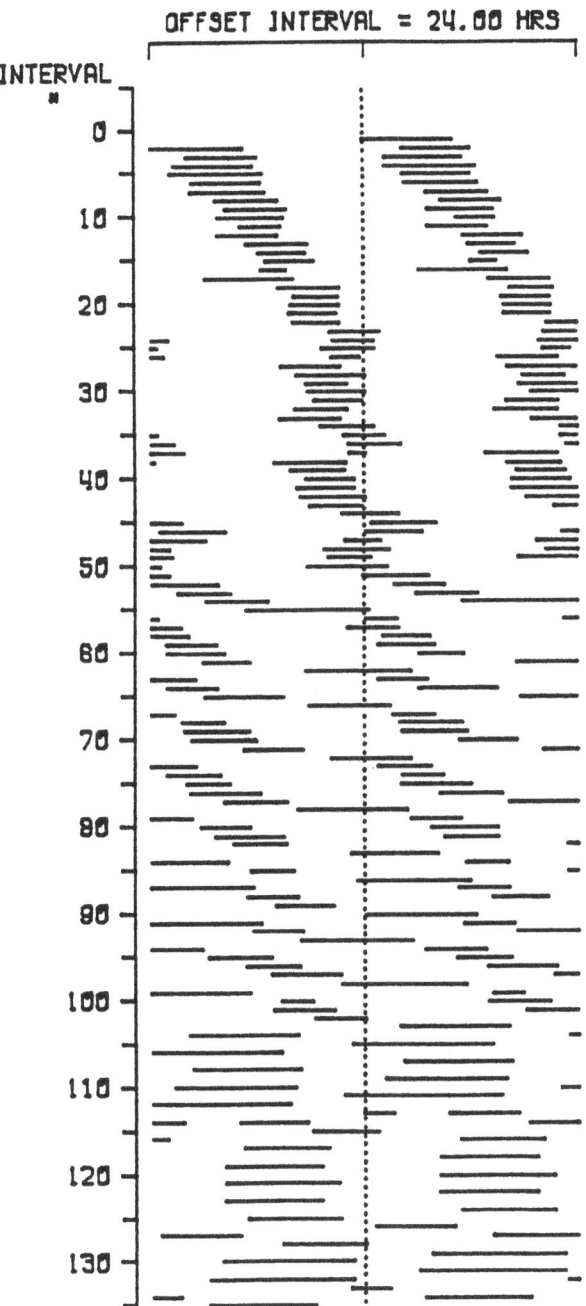

Figure 3-10. 24h raster plot for Subject 3.4.

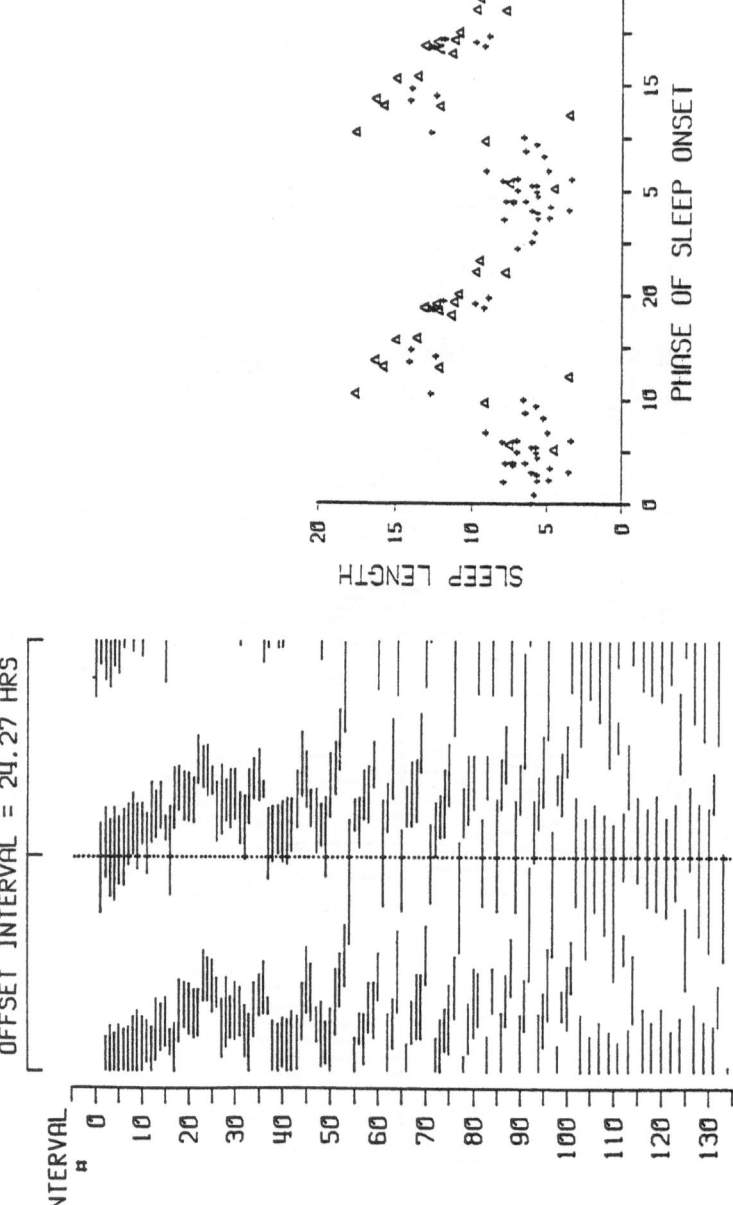

Figure 3-11. Normalized raster and sleep duration data for Subject 3.4.

3.5 Subject 5 (Siffre)

Remarks

This 6-month cave study was the grand finale of a series of experiments led by Michel Siffre in the late 60's and early 70's. Here, as in the pioneering study of 1962, Siffre was himself the subject. The sleep-wake record has been discussed already in Section 1.1.

The record contains some unusual phenomena. (1) Two desynchronies are separated by about two months of synchrony. (2) During that middle synchronized section, the compromise period varies on a 15-20 day time scale, a feature seen in no other record. (Modulations at that time scale were seen in LD03 (Figure 4-25), but they always led to desynchronized sleep-wake cycles.) (3) There is some indication that the circadian period τ may have changed from the first desynchrony to the second. But this is none too certain, since my methods are at the limits of their resolving power here. In any case, either of the choices for τ (25.3 or 25.6h) qualify as the longest ever observed. So does Siffre's compromise period of 26.4h.

I digitized the temperature minima (dots in Figure 3-13, left: top and bottom) and sleep data from xeroxed records in a document prepared by Siffre for the French government (obtained by C.A. Czeisler from M. Jouvet). One desynchrony (#1) is reported in Siffre's (1975) *National Geographic* article. Otherwise these wonderful data are nowhere to be found.

Statistics

	N	$\bar{\rho}$	$\bar{\alpha}$	F	τ_{SW}
synch	31	7.4	19.0	0.28	26.3±2.0
desynch #1	21	9.8	23.2	0.30	33.0±8.6
synch	58	7.9	18.6	0.30	26.4±2.9
desynch #2	16	10.4	25.0	0.29	35.5±6.1
phase-trap	13	7.9	19.5	0.29	27.5±5.6

τ estimate: 25.6 (1st desynch)
25.3 (2nd desynch)

temp. (minima)	sleep onsets	sleep length
25.65 (1st desynch)	25.6	25.55
25.30 (2nd desynch)	25.6	25.5

Sex	Age	Code	Source
M	33	MS	Siffre report to French government, 1977
			Siffre (1975)

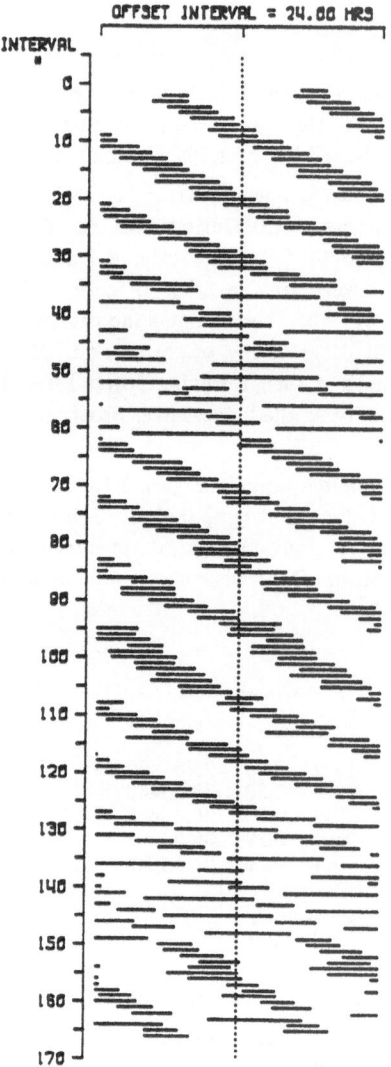

Figure 3-12. 24h raster plot for Subject 3.5.

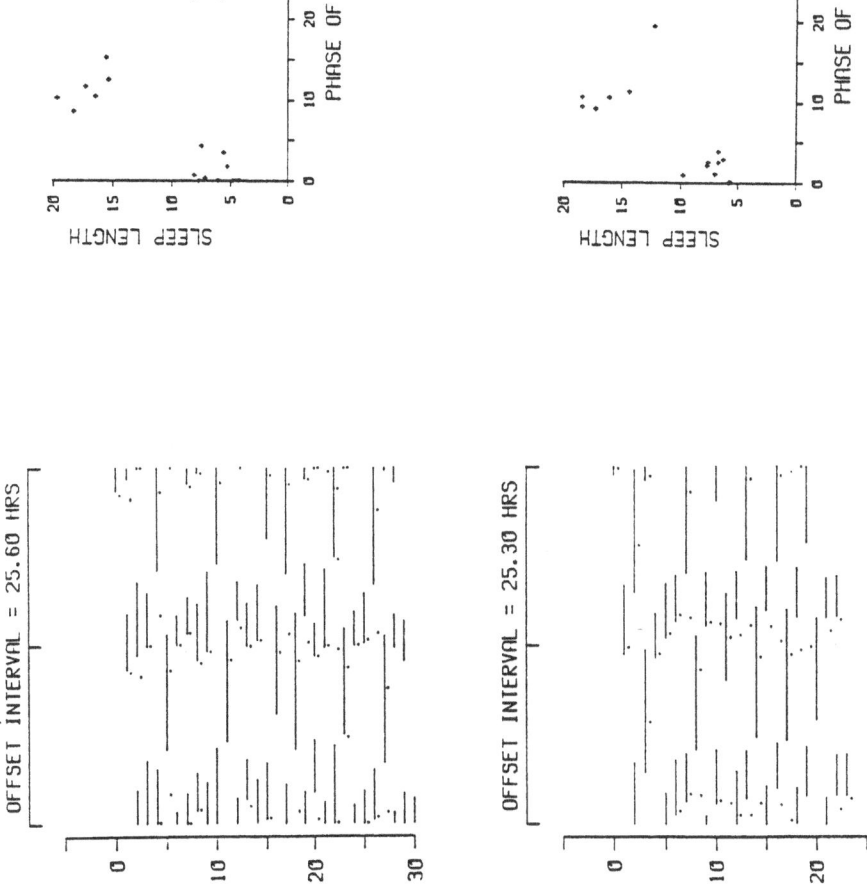

Figure 3-13. Normalized rasters and sleep duration data for Subject 3.5.

3.6 Subject 6 (Wever, Figure 36)

Remarks

This long record (43 cycles) from Wever (1979), Fig. 36 is of some theoretical interest. Daan *et al.* (1984) have tested their model by trying to simulate this record. They state (p. R169) that "the simulation and the real data correspond in considerable detail." I have not been able to reproduce their result (see Section 6.5.1 for reservations concerning other aspects of the published results of Daan *et al.* 1984).

The record in Wever (1979) shows a shortening of the temperature period, from a compromise period of 25.6h to a desynchronized value of 25.2h (cf. Section 4.9.1). Dots on the normalized raster (Figure 3-14) represent temperature minima.

Statistics

	N	$\bar{\rho}$	$\bar{\alpha}$	F	τ_{SW}
synch	26	8.0	17.7	0.31	25.8±2.7
desynch	17	9.9	19.3	0.34	29.1±4.8

τ estimate: 25.2

temperature	sleep onsets	sleep length
25.2	25.5	25.3

Sex	Age	Code	Source
M	26	KD	Wever, 1979 — Fig. 36
			Daan *et al.*, 1984 — Fig. 10A

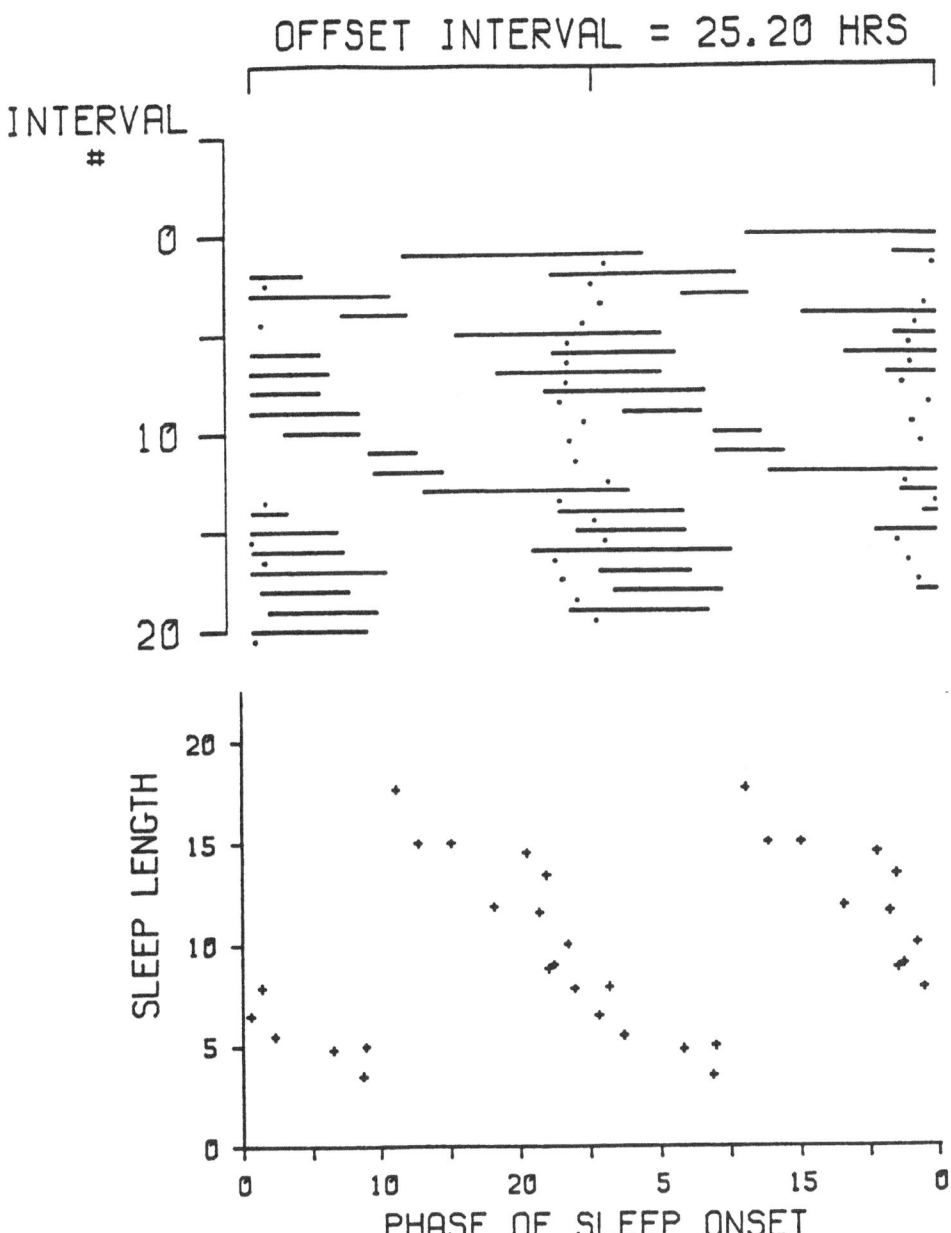

Figure 3-14. Normalized raster and sleep duration data for Subject 3.6.

3.7 Subject 7 (FR03)

Remarks

This 25 year old male was the first subject of Czeisler's (1978) study to exhibit internal desynchronization. His record exhibits phenomena of theoretical interest:

(1) gating of sleep onsets at certain circadian phases (cf. Section 4.4 and Figure 4-19).

(2) a monotonically increasing sleep-wake cycle period (cf. Section 4.8).

(3) a return of slow wave sleep during two long sleep episodes (cf. Section 5.4, Remark 2).

In Figure 3-15, reoccurrences of Stage 4 sleep are shown as heavy dark dots. (See Weitzman et al., 1979 for more information on this surprising phenomenon.)

Statistics

	N	$\bar{\rho}$	$\bar{\alpha}$	F	τ_{SW}
desynch	8	13.9	24.2	0.36	38.1±7.3

τ estimate: 25.08

temp.(eduction)	sleep onsets (1.5h bins)	sleep length
25.08	25.25	25.15

Sex	Age	Code	Source
M	25	FR03	Czeisler, 1978 — Fig. 14

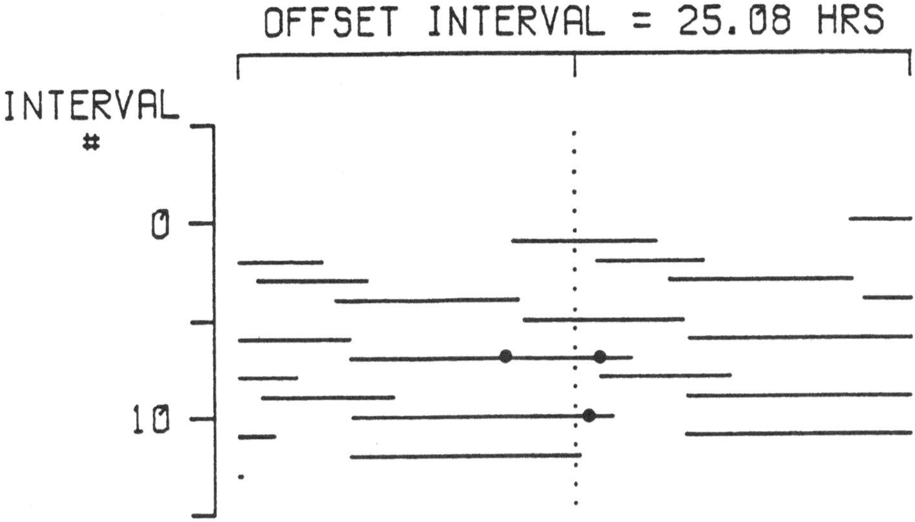

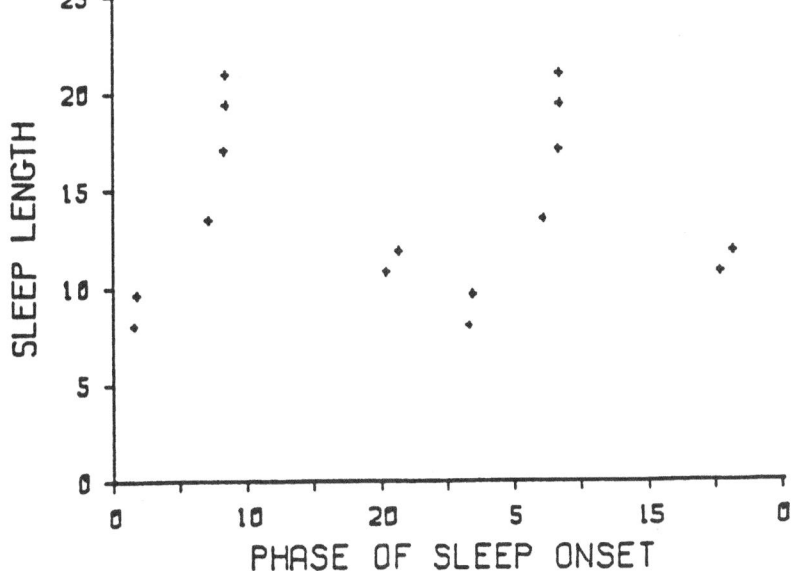

Figure 3-15. Normalized raster and sleep duration data for Subject 3.7. Filled circles, return of Stage 4 sleep.

3.8 Subject 8 (FR04)

Remarks

A 22 year old male, this subject provided the second case of desynchronization observed by Czeisler (1978).

The most unusual feature of this record is the length of the sleep episodes — all of them exceed the circadian phase-adjusted average values one would have expected, based on the $\phi_s{:}\rho$ relationship of Section 4.1.

Statistics

	N	$\bar{\rho}$	$\bar{\alpha}$	F	τ_{SW}
desynch	9	13.4	23.6	0.36	37.0±4.0

τ estimate: 24.33

temp. (eduction)	Sleep onsets	Sleep length
24.33	24.30	24.7

Sex	Age	Code	Source
M	22	FR04	Czeisler, 1978 — Fig. 14

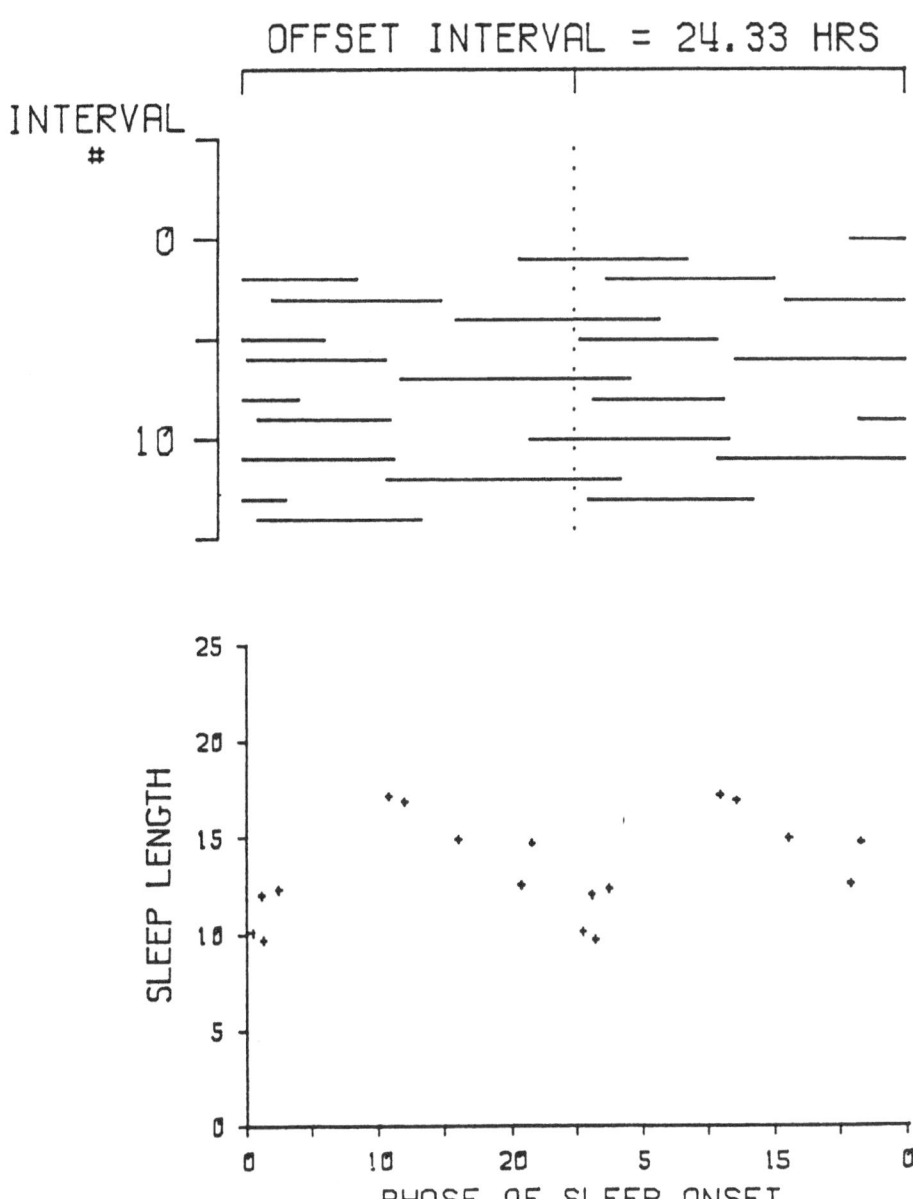

Figure 3-16. Normalized raster and sleep duration data for Subject 3.8.

3.9 Subject 9 (FR10)

Remarks

This subject was a retired fireman. Like other subjects in Czeisler's experiments he was asked to assess his alertness at frequent intervals during his waking day. When asked why he invariably assessed himself as being "very alert" he said that he was always ready for a fire!

His record is especially interesting because of his peculiar entrained circadian phase: in the outside world he was probably taking his nocturnal sleep episode *before* the evening wake-maintenance zone (Section 4.5), near the circadian *nap* phase. In other words, his temperature trough was located near noon (Figure 3-17, dashed line), an astonishing time for a 51 year old. The possibility of stable entrainment at this internal phase relationship is problematic for all the available models (which typically predict only one stable phase position for sleep, about 180° opposite nap phase).

His circadian phase position has been estimated by (1) temperature eduction during entrainment and free-run, (2) comparison with the sleep duration-circadian phase curve, (3) location of those sleep episodes with short REM latency (time from lights out to mid-REM < 30 minutes). Such short REM latency occurs in normal subjects only when sleep begins near the temperature trough (Czeisler, 1978; Czeisler *et al.*, 1980a,b; Carskadon and Dement, 1980). Episodes with REM onset are indicated by small open circles in Figure 3-18. All three estimates point to the interpretations above.

Statistics

	N	$\bar{\rho}$	$\bar{\alpha}$	F	τ_{SW}
desynch	12	11.8	28.0	0.30	39.8±6.5

τ estimate: 24.27

temp. (eduction)	sleep onsets	sleep length
24.27	24.35	24.35

Sex	Age	Code	Source
M	51	FR10	Czeisler, 1978 — Fig. 15 Kronauer *et al.*, 1983 — Fig. 2

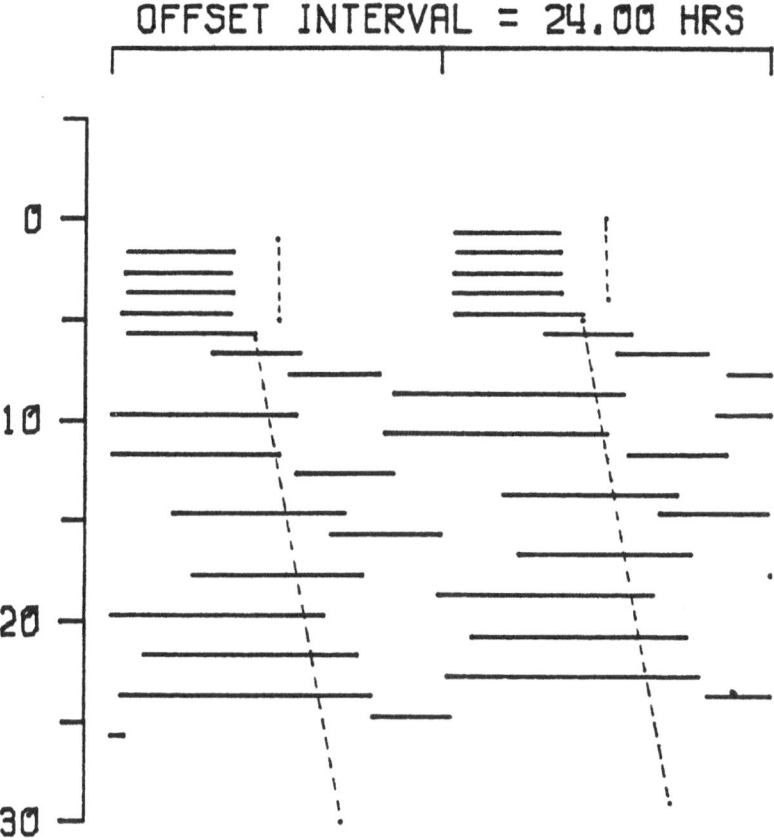

Figure 3-17. 24h raster plot for Subject 3.9. Dashed lines, educed mid-low temperature.

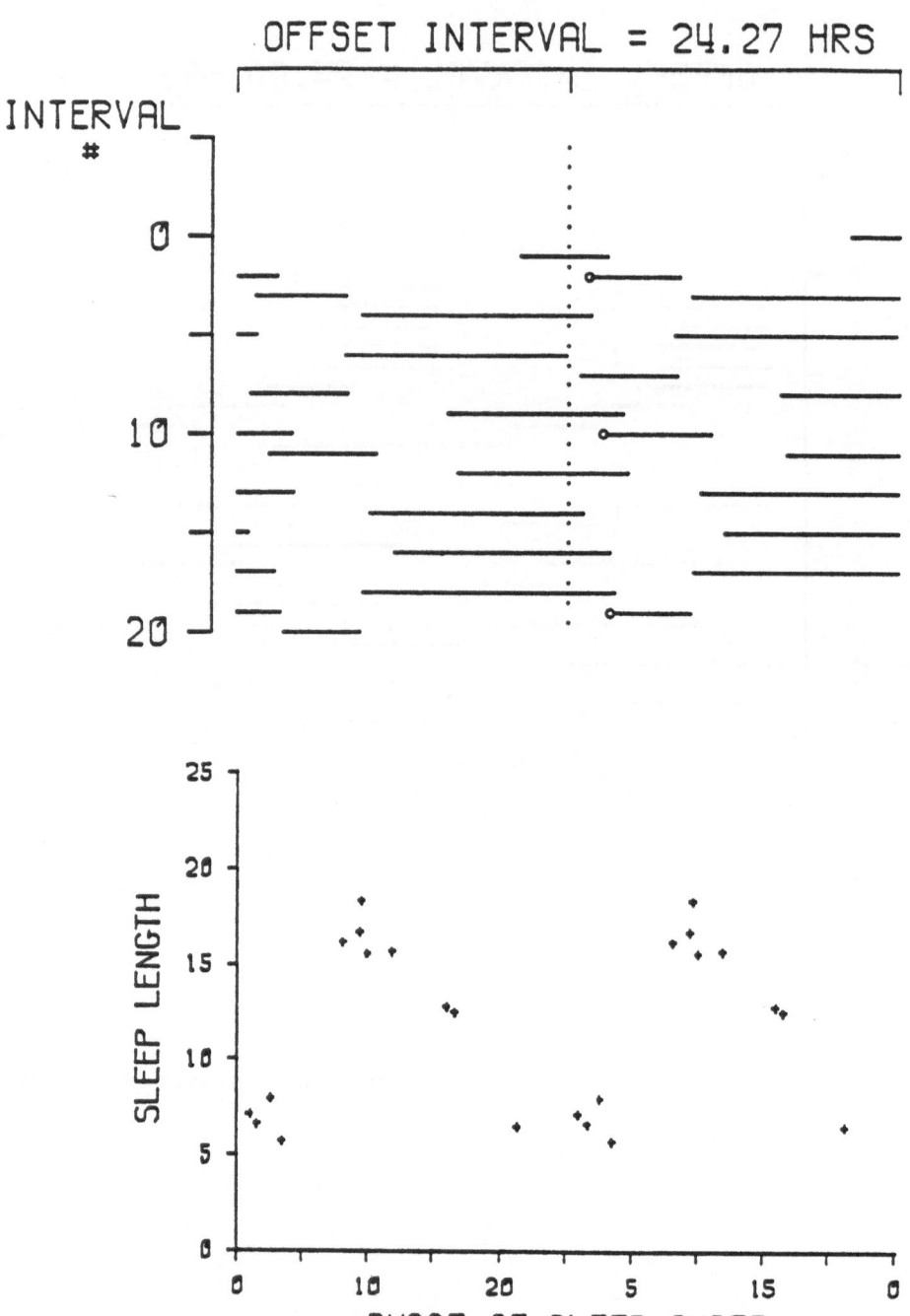

Figure 3-18. Normalized raster and sleep duration data for Subject 3.9. Open circles, sleep onset REM episodes.

3.10 Subject 10 (Aschoff, 1965)

Remarks

This record is the first published example of spontaneous internal desynchronization, reported in 1965 by Aschoff. All the main patterns discussed in Chapter 4 — wake-maintenance zones, dependence of sleep length on circadian phase, etc. — are present in this first example of desynchrony.

The first two sleep episodes of the original record have been omitted here; they appear to be part of a transient adjustment of internal phase after release from entrainment. On the normalized raster, dots represent temperature *maxima* (Figure 3-19).

Statistics

	N	$\bar{\rho}$	$\bar{\alpha}$	F	τ_{SW}
synch	2	8.7	18.9	0.32	27.6±1.8
desynch	17	10.7	21.7	0.33	32.4±5.6

τ estimate: 24.5

temperature	sleep onsets	sleep duration
24.4	24.4	24.7
24.7 (Aschoff)		

Sex	Age	Code	Source
N/A	N/A	N/A	Aschoff, 1965 — Fig. 7
			Moore-Ede *et al.*, 1982 — Fig. 3.12

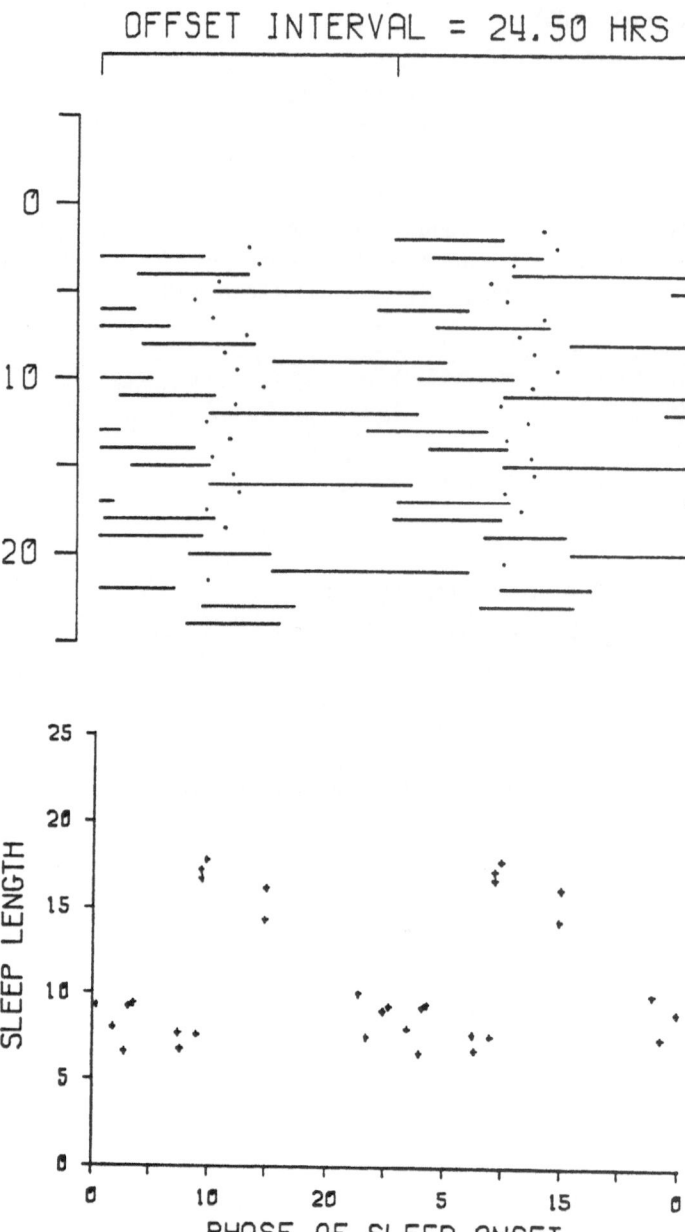

Figure 3-19. Normalized raster and sleep duration data for Subject 3.10. Dots, temperature maxima.

3.11 Subject 11 (Aschoff, 1969)

Remark

An early example of internal desynchronization reported by Aschoff (1969). Dots on the normalized raster (Figure 3-20) represent temperature minima.

Statistics

	N	$\bar{\rho}$	$\bar{\alpha}$	F	τ_{SW}
synch	6	9.9	14.9	0.40	24.9±1.6
desynch	11	11.7	20.0	0.37	31.8±4.6

τ estimate: 24.9

temp. (minima)	Sleep onsets	Sleep length
24.9	25.15	24.7

Sex	Age	Code	Source
N/A	N/A	N/A	Aschoff, 1969 — Fig. 5

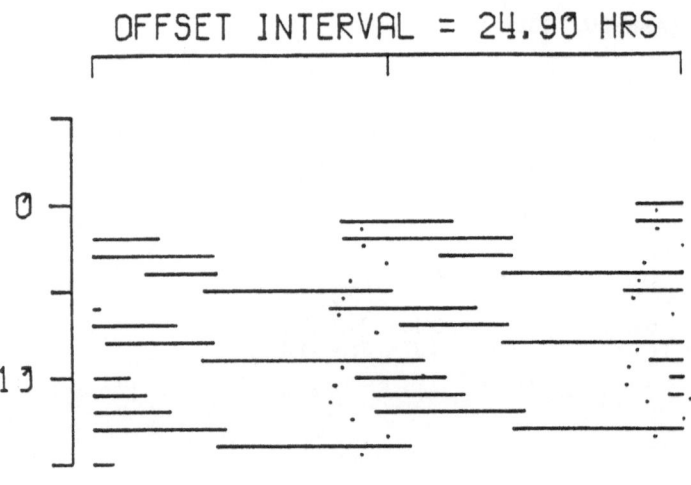

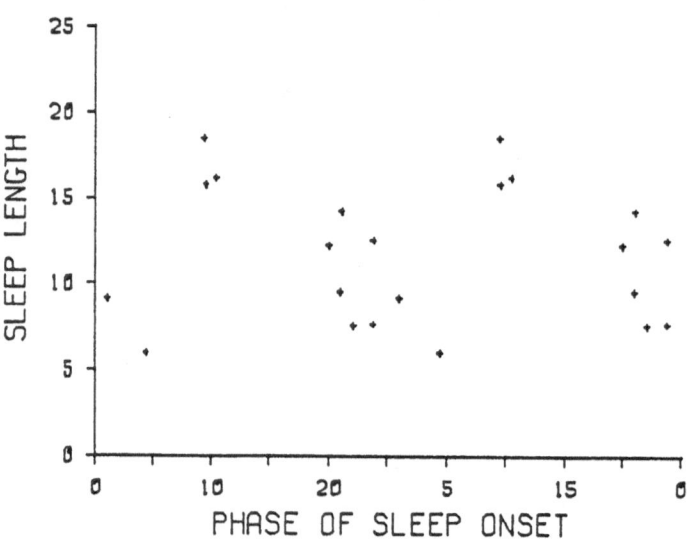

Figure 3-20. Normalized raster and sleep duration data for Subject 3.11. Dots, approximate temperature minima.

3.12 Subject 12 (Wever, Figure 27)

Remarks

This record is often shown in publications of Wever, Zulley, and Aschoff, just as PR01 is the exemplary record for Czeisler's group.

The original record nicely shows the shortening of the temperature period after internal desynchronization, from 25.7h to 25.1h. In this respect too the record is like PR01.

Dots on the normalized raster (Figure 3-21) locate temperature minima.

Statistics

	N	$\bar{\rho}$	$\bar{\alpha}$	F	τ_{SW}
synch	11	7.1	18.5	0.28	25.6±2.2
desynch	15	9.2	24.0	0.28	33.1±4.2

τ estimate: 25.1

temperature	Sleep onsets	Sleep length
25.1	25.2	25.5

Sex	Age	Code	Source
F	24	EvS	Wever, 1979 — Fig. 27
			Wever, 1975 — p. 36
			Zulley *et al.*, 1981 — Fig. 1
			Eastman, 1984 — Fig. 1

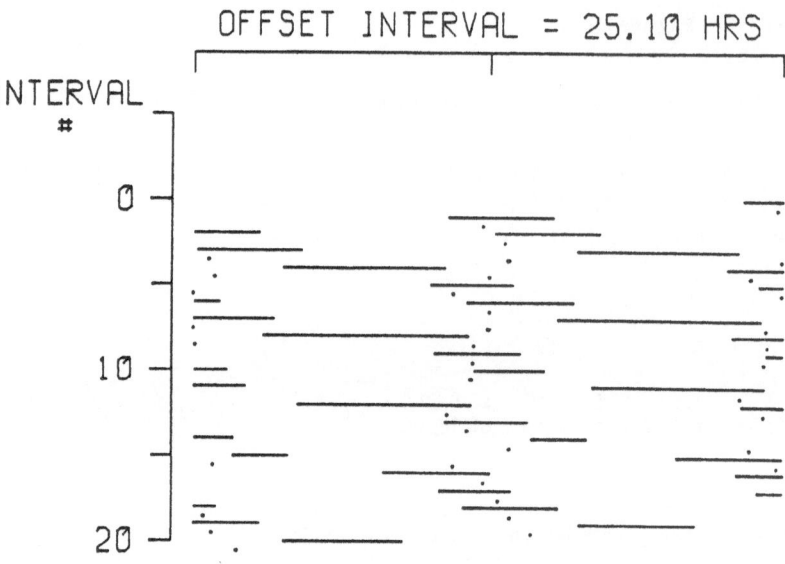

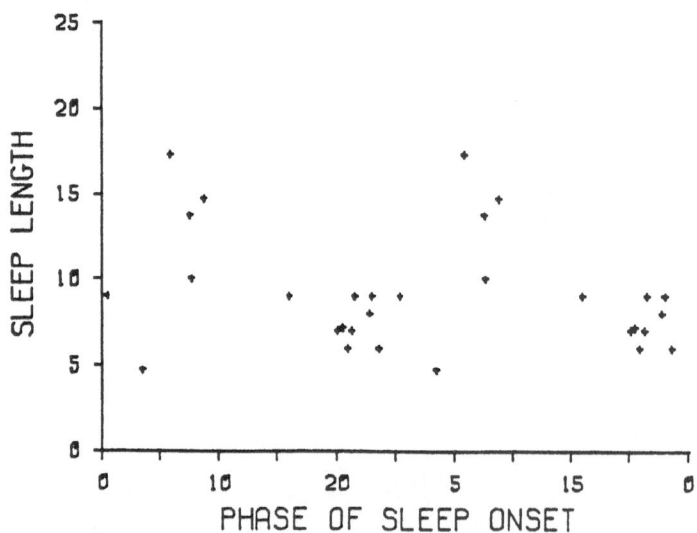

Figure 3-21. Normalized raster and sleep duration data for Subject 3.12. Dots, temperature minima.

3.13 Subject 13 (Aschoff *et al.*, 1967)

Remarks

The temperature estimates here seem unreliable. Data were presented by Aschoff *et al.*, 1967 as temperature waveforms on an activity raster plot. I have estimated the minimum of each temperature cycle by eye (dots on Figure 3-22), but there may be considerable error here. Sleep-wake data were also used to estimate circadian period and phase by the methods described in Section 4.6.

Statistics

N	$\bar{\rho}$	$\bar{\alpha}$	F	τ_{SW}
16	12.3	20.8	0.37	33.1±5.1

τ estimate: 24.7

temperature	sleep onsets	sleep length
24.8	24.3 (major peak) 24.7 (minor peak)	24.7

Sex	Age	Code	Source
N/A	N/A	F	Aschoff *et al.*, 1967 — Fig. 4

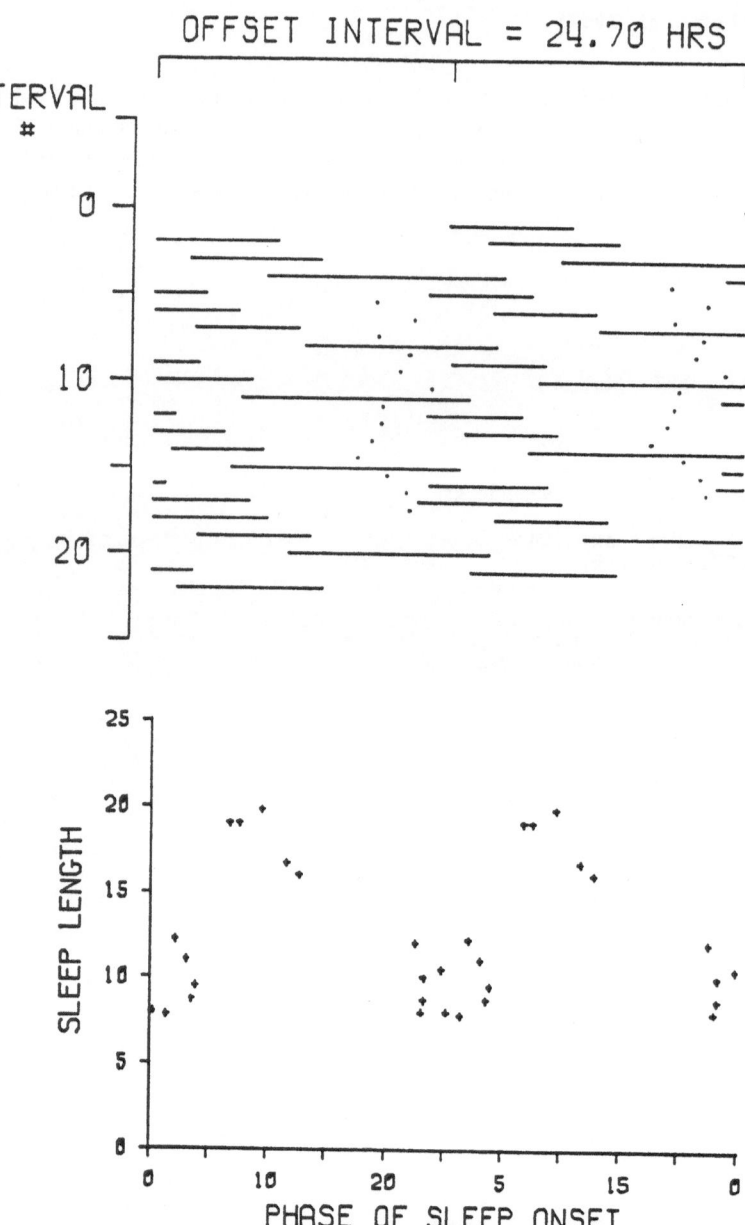

Figure 3-22. Normalized raster and sleep duration data for Subject 3.13. Dots, approximate temperature minima.

3.14 Subject 14 (Mills G6)

Remarks

The only temperature data reported were local maxima (dots on Figure 3-23).

The sleep-wake study here was performed in an isolation unit, and the sleep data are more believable than those of the cave study also reported by Mills *et al.* (Section 3.16) in the same paper.

Statistics

N	$\bar{\rho}$	$\bar{\alpha}$	F	τ_{SW}
8	11.7	23.1	0.34	34.8±6.3

τ estimate: 25.1

temp. (maxima)		sleep onsets	sleep length
25.1		25.1	25.0-25.5 (flat minimum)

Sex	Age	Code	Source
M	19	G6	Mills *et al.*, 1974 — Fig. 4

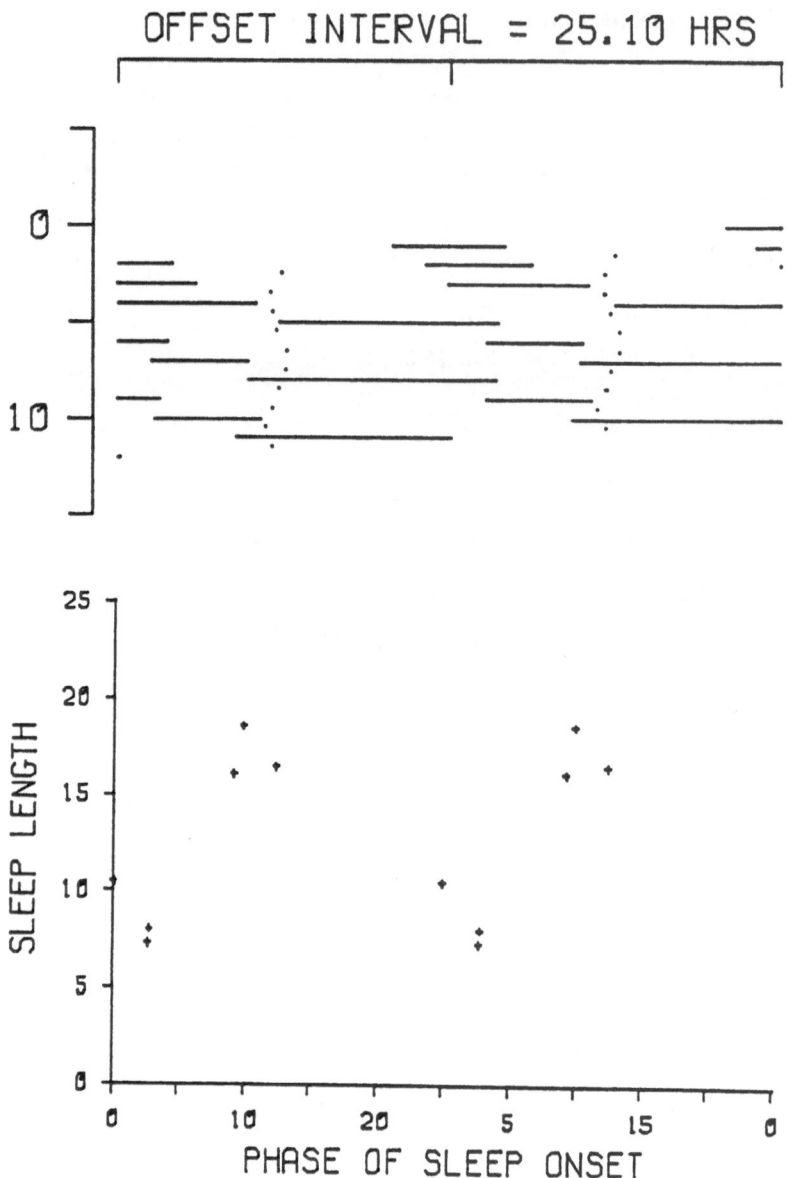

Figure 3-23. Normalized raster and sleep duration data for Subject 3.14. Dots, temperature maxima.

3.15 Subject 15 (Wever, Figure 54)

Remarks

Wever (1979, p. 101) maintains that DC electric or magnetic fields "are neither able to affect the autonomous period nor to prevent internal desynchronization." Therefore, although an artificial electric field was on during the time when this subject desynchronized, it is probably safe to ignore it. The sleep-wake record looks like that of other desynchronized subjects (e.g., Subject 3.7).

The three long sleeps are among the longest ever observed (20.3, 22.3, and 18.2h, respectively). Since there was no EEG recording, it is possible that the subject lay awake in bed for some of the time. Yet given the circadian phases of those sleep onsets, it is conceivable that the subject really did sleep that long — compare e.g., FR03 (Section 3.7) or 426F (Section 3.3), for whom EEGs were recorded.

In synchrony and desynchrony, the subject had a high sleep fraction of 0.39.

Statistics

	N	$\bar{\rho}$	$\bar{\alpha}$	F	τ_{SW}
synch	11	10.1	15.8	0.39	25.9 ± 3.2
desynch	7	14.0	21.9	0.39	35.9 ± 5.4

τ estimate: 24.9

temperature	sleep onsets	sleep duration
24.9	24.9	25.1

Sex	Age	Code	Source
M	27	HN	Wever, 1979 — Fig. 54

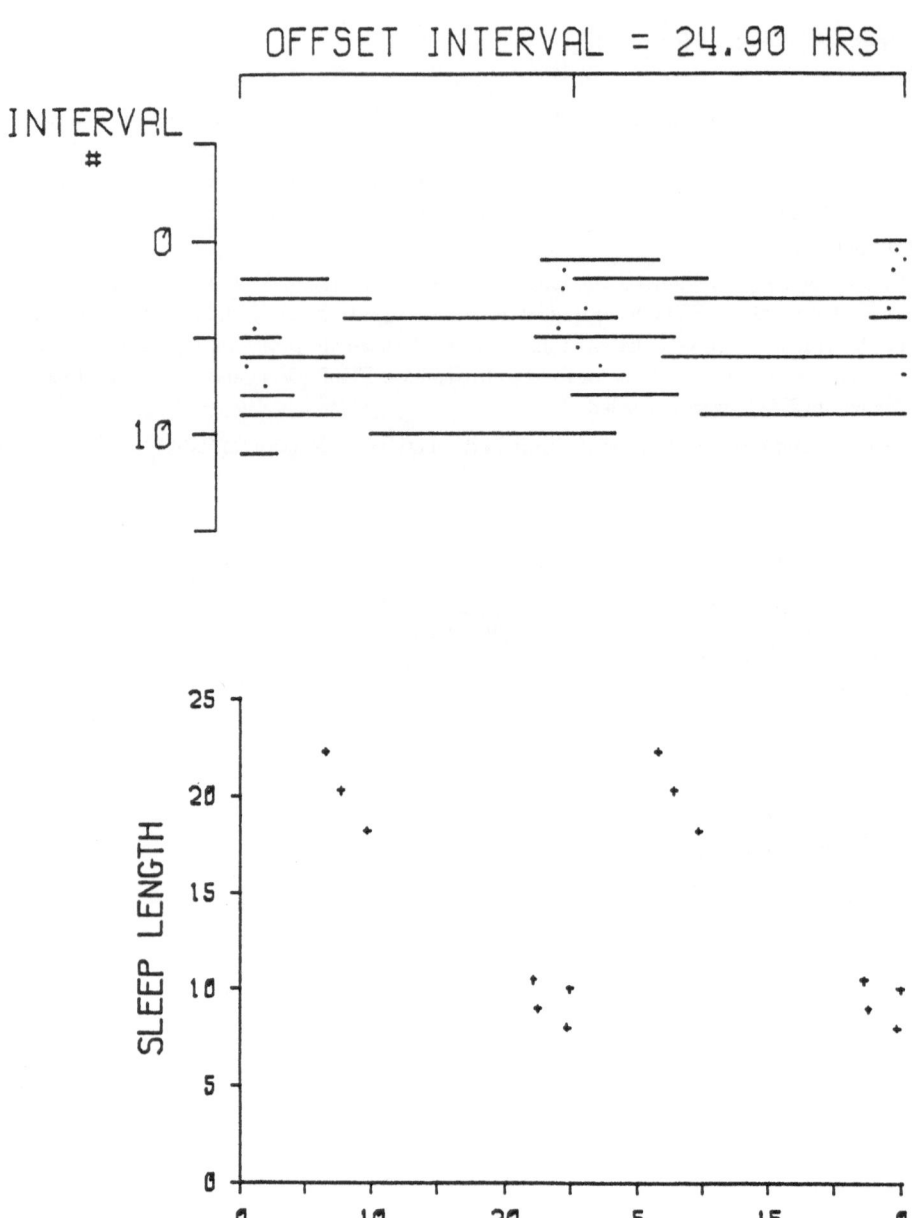

Figure 3-24. Normalized raster and sleep duration data for Subject 3.15. Dots, temperature minima.

3.16 Subject 16 (Mills DL)

Remarks

This record of a 4-month cave study should be viewed with some caution. The nominal "sleep episodes" are actually times in bed (Winfree, 1983). There is reason to doubt that the subject was asleep throughout the bedrest — in some instances he stayed in bed for more than 35h, and his "sleep" fraction exceeds 0.6! These numbers are unheard of in any subject for whom sleep was polygraphically verified. No doubt many of the bedrests were punctuated with hours of wakefulness.

So what conclusions about sleep may be drawn from this record of bedrest? Probably the times of retiring reliably mark sleep onsets, whereas the times of rising may have little to do with true awakening. Based on the bedrest onsets (Figure 3-25), it appears that the subject was internally desynchronized after day 5, and then spontaneously synchronized around day 45. Occasional "out of phase" sleeps occur until around day 75, after which synchrony is maintained (except near day 115).

The circadian period was estimated by considering sleep-wake cycles 5-21, the most desynchronized portion of the record (Figure 3-26). A period of 24.87h gave maximum clustering of sleep onsets (cf. Section 4.6). Circadian phase was estimated by replotting the data at this period. Two wake-maintenance zones appeared, and their phases were consistent with those estimated from the sleep length data.

Note that the sleep-wake period gradually shortened during this experiment (cf. Section 4.8).

Winfree (1983) offered a different interpretation of this record. Based on the zone of forbidden wake-ups (Section 4.3), he postulated that the circadian period τ drifts from 24.5h to 25.3 over the 4 months of temporal isolation. Such a dramatic drift cannot be ruled out, but it seems unlikely; compare Subjects 3.2, 3.4, and 3.5 in whom the circadian periods are stable to within about 1%.

Statistics

	N	$\bar{\rho}$	$\bar{\alpha}$	F	τ_{SW}
synch	4	17.5	8.6	0.67	26.1±1.4
desynch	41	21.6	13.3	0.62	34.9±9.8
synch	56	15.7	10.6	0.60	26.3±3.5

τ estimate: 24.87

temperature	sleep onsets	sleep length
N/A	24.87	24.6-24.9

Sex	Age	Code	Source
M	28	DL	Mills *et al.*, 1974 — Fig. 8 Winfree, 1983 — Fig. 6

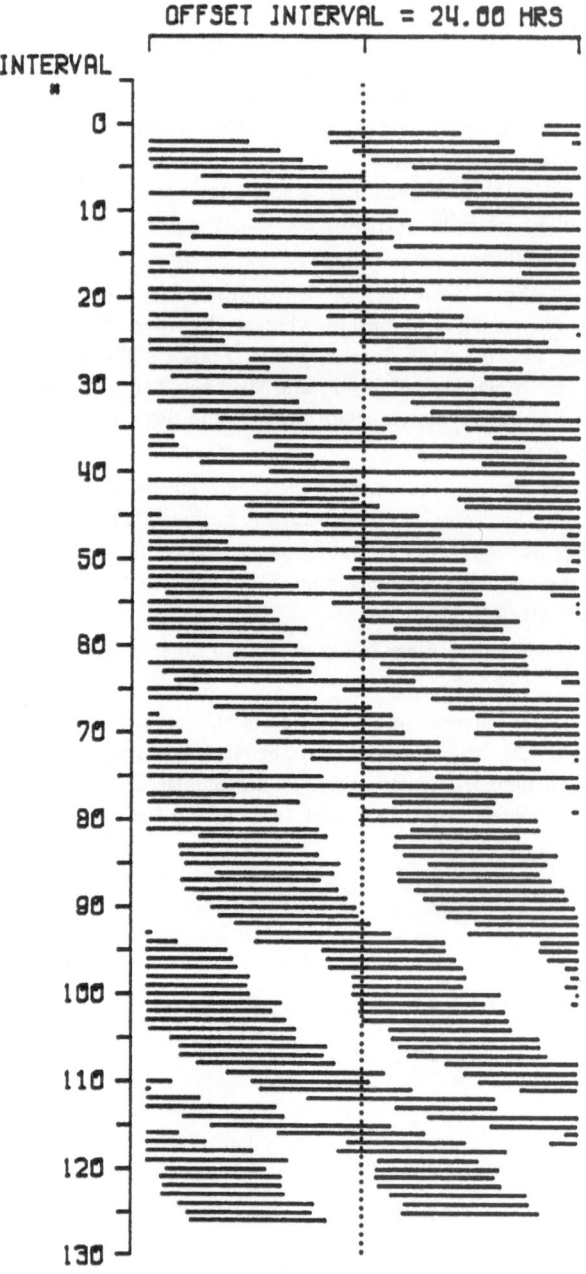

Figure 3-25. 24h raster plot for Subject 3.16.

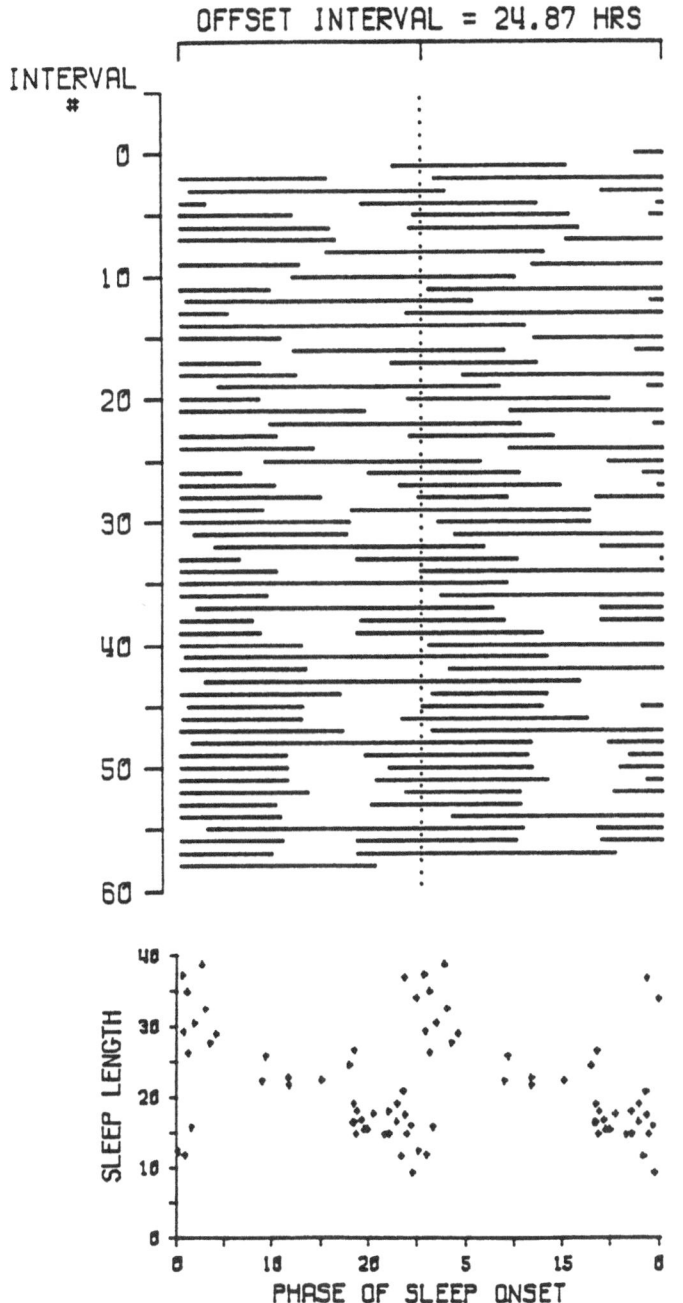

Figure 3-26. Normalized raster and sleep duration data for Subject 3.16.

3.17 Subject 17 (LD04)

Remarks

This subject is unusual in that he remained internally synchronized for more than 4 months of free-run. All other subjects free-running for longer than 2 months have spontaneously desynchronized at some time (Czeisler, 1978; Czeisler et al., 1980a).

But the conditions preceding free-run were unusual too. In a light-dark entrainment study, he lived for 20 cycles on an enforced 24h schedule, then for 21 cycles on a 25h schedule, and then back to 13 more cycles of 24h.

It has been suggested (Kronauer et al., 1982) that prior entrainment to 25h could have lengthened the subject's intrinsic circadian period, thus hindering desynchronization. Such "aftereffects" on free-running period are known to last one hundred days or more in some animals (Pittendrigh and Daan, 1976; Moore-Ede et al., 1982, Figure 2.7).

Note that between days 85–115 there is some indication of phase-trapping with a cycle of ∼ 5 days. This is the closest the subject came to desynchrony and it occurs near the end of the experiment.

Statistics

N	$\overline{\rho}$	$\overline{\alpha}$	F	τ_{SW}
121	9.2	16.0	0.37	25.2±2.5

Sex	Age	Code	Source
M	24	LD04	Unpublished (but see footnote, Kronauer et al., 1982, p. R3)

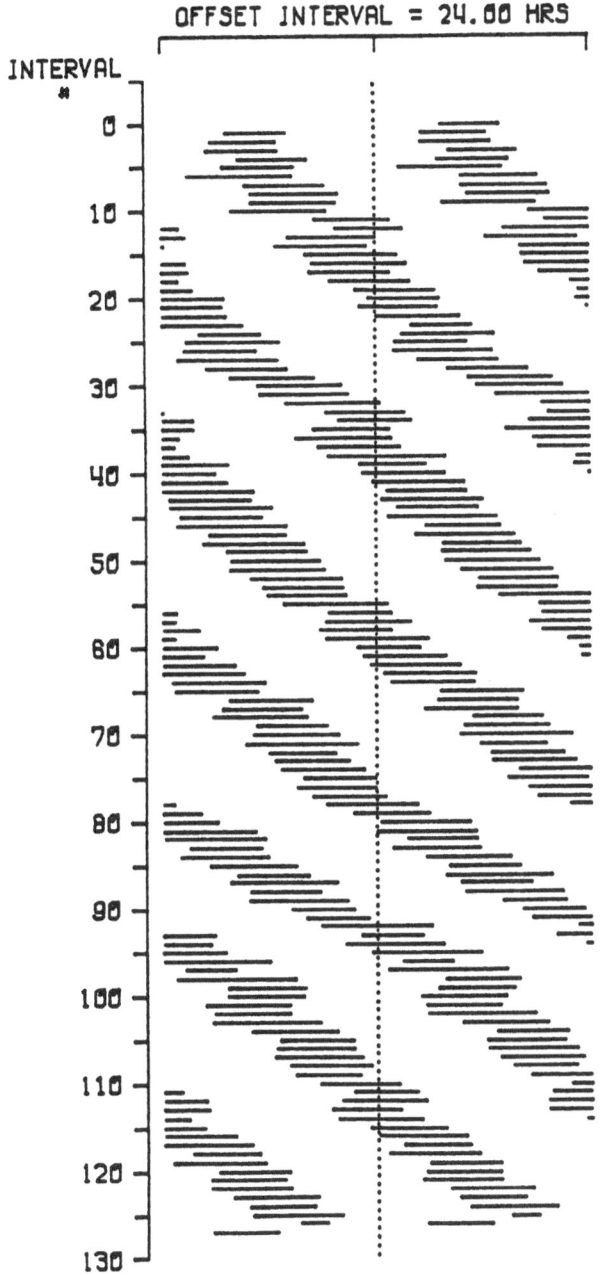

Figure 3-27. 24h raster plot for Subject 3.17.

3.18 Subject 18 (FR11)

Remarks

FR11 was an 81 year old male who habitually napped. Along with Subject 3.19 and Subject 3.20, he was participating in a study of napping during free-run.

The circadian period of 24.05h was estimated by considering sleep onset clustering and the location of the wake-maintenance zones. Because of its low amplitude, the temperature rhythm seemed a less reliable estimator of period (estimate $\tau = 24.37$h). However, temperature data were educed at $\tau = 24.05$, with mid-low temperature at phase 0.

There is consistency between FR11 and FR19 (Subject 3.19), with regard to the sleep length vs. phase data. The curves align in phase, although FR11 has several long sleeps which are absent from FR19's record.

Statistics

N	$\bar{\rho}$	$\bar{\alpha}$	F	τ_{SW}
36	4.1	9.3	0.31	13.3±3.2

τ estimate: 24.05

temp. (eduction)	sleep onsets	sleep length
24.37	24.05 & 24.25	24.14

Sex	Age	Code	Source
M	81	FR11	Weitzman *et al.*, unpublished data (but see Weitzman *et al.*, 1982)

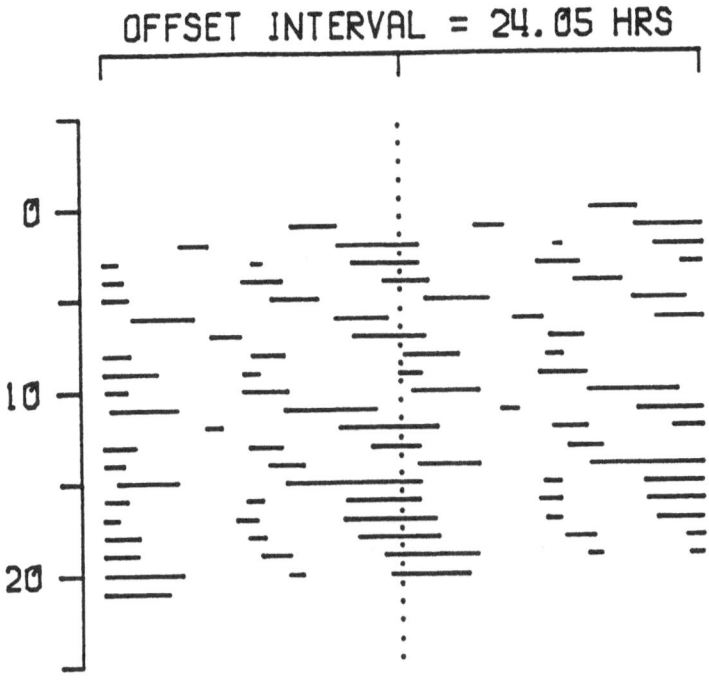

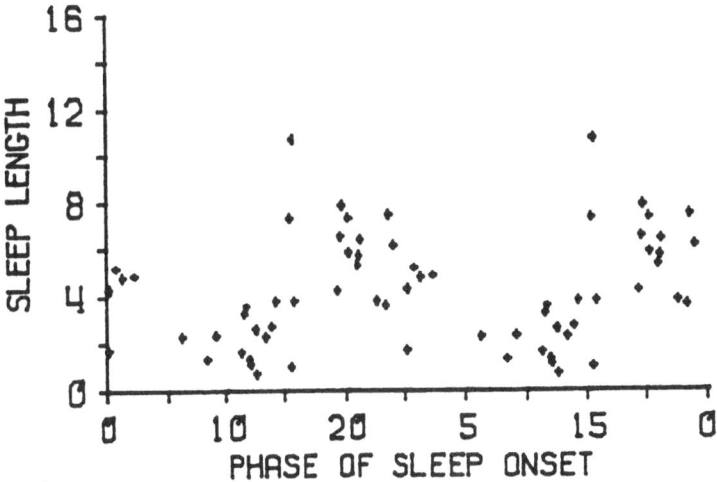

Figure 3-28. Normalized raster and sleep duration data for Subject 3.18.

3.19 Subject 19 (FR19)

Remarks

The subject was a 67 male who habitually napped. Along with FR11 (Subject 3.18) and FR20 (Subject 3.20), he was participating in a study of napping during free-run.

For this record, as well as for FR11, the period from temperature eduction has not been used as the estimate of τ. Napping tends to worsen evoked effects, and in any case the period indicated by eduction was part of a broad minimum, with little to choose from.

A circadian period $\tau \sim 24.6$ was estimated on several grounds: (1) It yields wake-maintenance zones at the expected phases. (2) It produces a tight relation between sleep length and circadian phase. (3) When the subject was re-entrained at the end of the experiment, his temperature record consistently showed local minima before his scheduled nap. (Such minima never occurred during entrainment at the beginning of the experiment.) The anomalous minima probably represent the actual trough of the circadian temperature rhythm, as they occur at the phase extrapolated from the hypothesized 24.6h rhythm. In other words, the subject appears to have been re-entrained such that *he was napping at low temperature*, 180° opposite from his usual circadian nap phase! (4) To check this, it was noted that he had REM during all of his re-entrained naps, whereas he had REM only once in his five naps during prior entrainment. This observation suggests that he was napping near the circadian trough, the phase of peak REM propensity (Czeisler *et al*, 1980a,b).

Statistics

N	$\bar{\rho}$	$\bar{\alpha}$	F	τ_{SW}
28	2.9	10.6	0.22	13.5±3.4

τ estimate: 24.60

Temperature	sleep onsets	sleep length
24.15	24.50	24.3-24.65

Sex	Age	Code	Source
M	67	FR19	Weitzman *et al.*, unpublished data Weitzman *et al.*, 1982

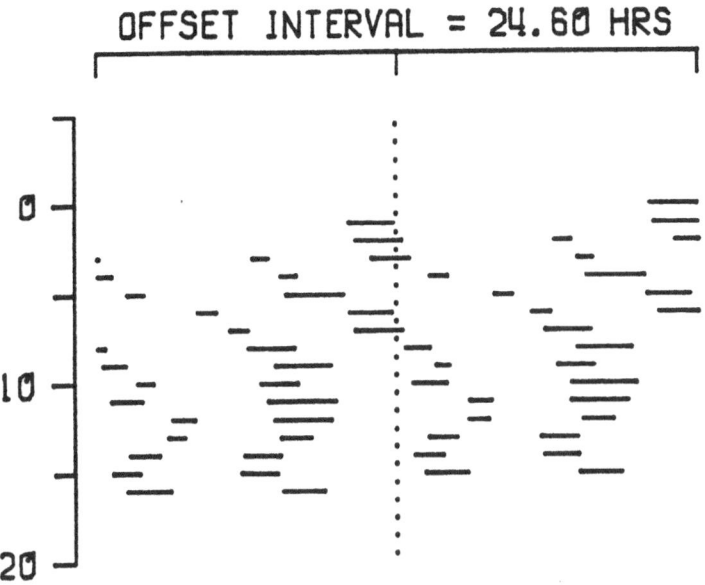

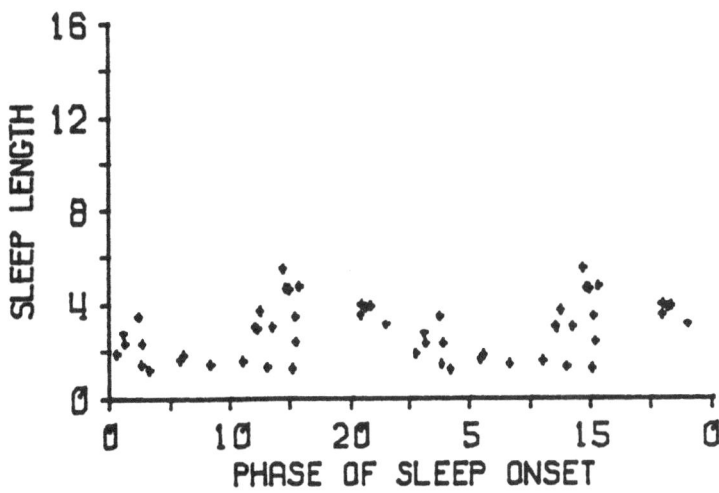

Figure 3-29. Normalized raster and sleep duration data for Subject 3.19.

3.20 Subject 20 (FR20)

Remarks

FR20 was participating in a study of napping during free-run, along with FR11 (Subject 3.18) and FR19 (Subject 3.19). Whereas those subjects were old men who habitually napped, FR20 was a 24 year-old man who did not nap in the outside world, but was entrained to a nap schedule for a week in the laboratory.

His free-running sleep-wake record, like that of Subjects 3.21 and 3.22, showed occasional splitting of the major sleep episode into two smaller sleep episodes: a nap ($\sim$ 3h) and a sleep ($\sim$ 5h). On other days his sleep was consolidated into one episode. He did not internally desynchronize in the usual sense. As such it is difficult to estimate his circadian phase, because the temperature cycle is heavily masked by the activity rhythm that is synchronized to it. For simplicity the mid-trough of the educed temperature waveform was chosen as phase 0, recognizing the limitations of this assessment. A second possibility, using $\tau = 24.72$, slightly widens the wake-maintenance zones and is shown in Figure 4-29 (Section 4.10).

Statistics

N	$\bar{\rho}$	$\bar{\alpha}$	F	τ_{SW}
42	6.1	12.5	0.33	18.6±5.7

τ estimate: 24.68

temp. (eduction)	sleep onsets	sleep length
24.68	24.65 or 24.80	24.7

Sex	Age	Code	Source
M	24	FR20	Weitzman et al., 1982

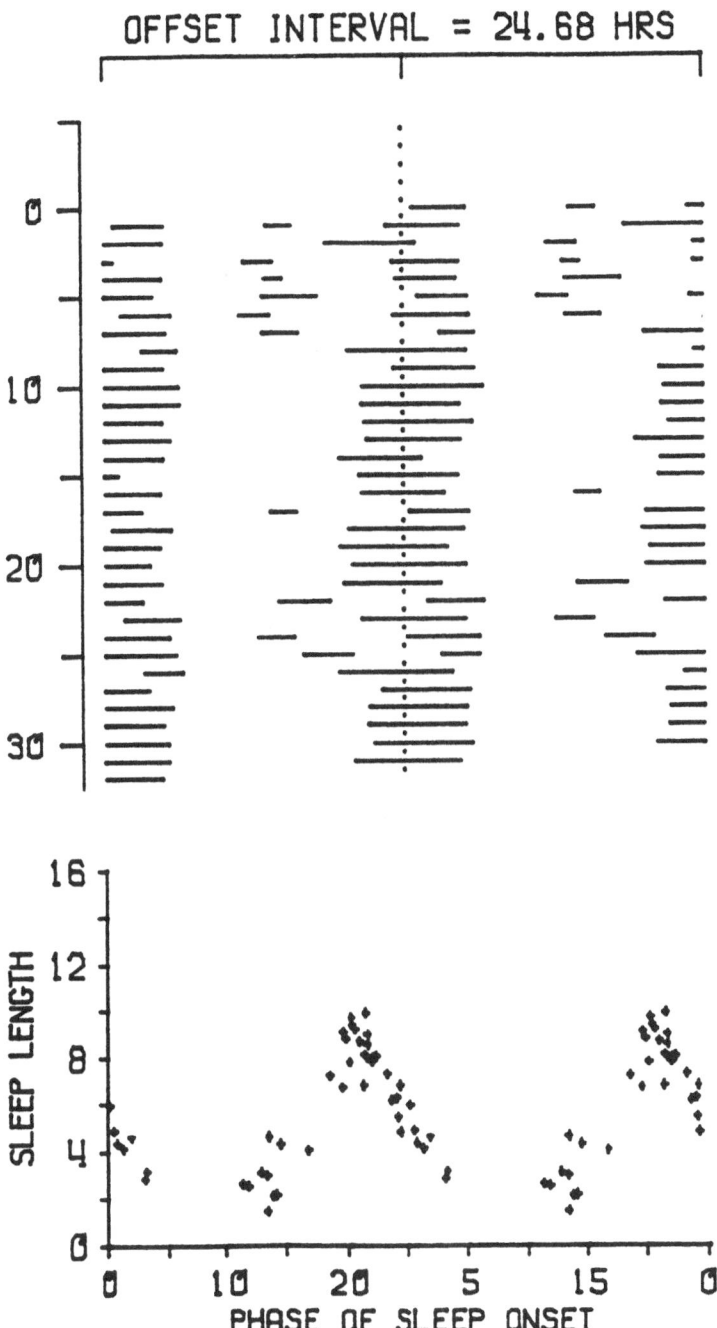

Figure 3-30. Normalized raster and sleep duration data for Subject 3.20.

3.21 Subject 21 (Wever, Figure 33)

Remarks

An example of split sleep, similar to Subject 3.20 and Subject 3.22. The record was plotted by Wever (1979) as an "apparent internal desynchronization" with short sleep-wake period, and interpreted by him as an example of 1:2 synchronization between activity and temperature cycles.

Sleep episodes 1-9 and 12-15 were split, while episodes 10-11 and 16-24 were consolidated. The subject apparently moved easily between split and consolidated regimes. During split sleep the naps averaged 3.4h and the sleeps averaged 4.8h. Wever (1979) comments that during the split episodes "the subject did not perceive the abnormal shortness of her activity time which averaged only 8.0 hours. During these short intervals, she took mostly three meals."

Of theoretical interest: split sleep can occur for several cycles in a row — whereas simulations with the Daan *et al.* (1984) model can give splitting, but only in a strict alternation with consolidated sleeps (cf. Section 7.2).

Statistics

N	$\bar{\rho}$	$\bar{\alpha}$	F	τ_{SW}
25	7.1	10.8	0.40	17.9$\pm$6.4

τ estimate: 24.39

temperature		sleep onsets	sleep length
24.5		24.4	24.2

Sex	Age	Code	Source
F	20	M.B.	Wever, 1979 — Fig. 33

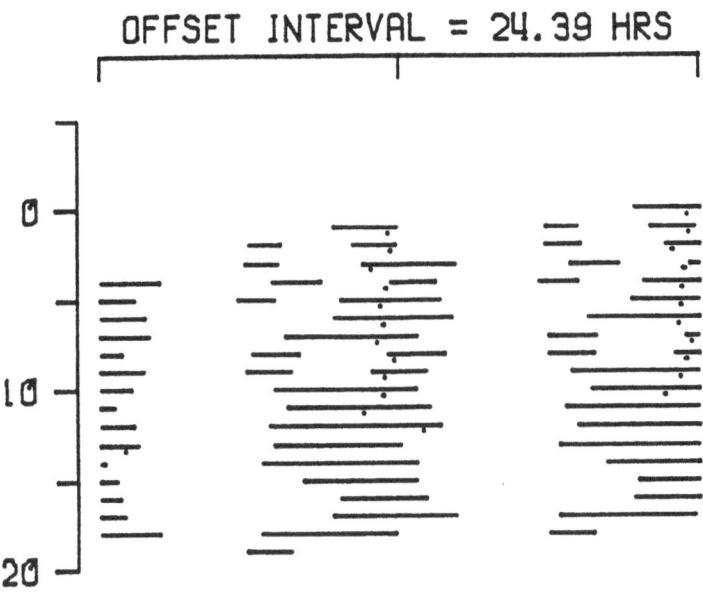

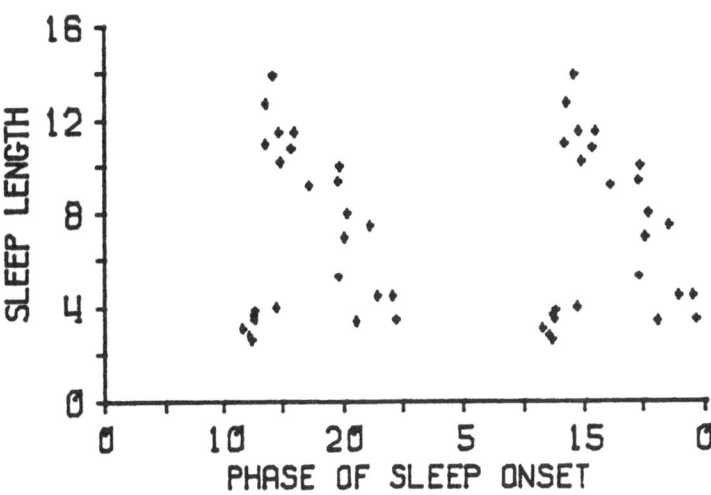

Figure 3-31. Normalized raster and sleep duration data for Subject 3.21.

3.22 Subject 22 (Wever, Figure 59)

Remarks

An example of split sleep, similar to FR20 (Subject 3.20) and Wever, Figure 33 (Subject 3.21). The subject alternates between a few consolidated sleeps in a row, and a pair of short sleep episodes. As in subjects 3.20 and 3.21, during split sleep the "naps" averaged 3.5h. Yet the "sleeps" were shorter (3.1h vs. 5h) for this subject, because they occurred at such a delayed circadian phase. In the last five sleep-wake cycles, an artificial electric field (10 Hz, AC, 2.5 V/m) was switched on — Wever attributes the consolidation at the end of the record to the influence of this electric field. Such an explanation may be superfluous, given the similarity of this record to others where no AC field was present.

Statistics

N	$\bar{\rho}$	$\bar{\alpha}$	F	τ_{SW}
25	6.8	13.4	0.34	20.2±3.8

τ estimate: 24.20

temperature	sleep onsets	sleep length
24.25	24.10	24.1–24.3

Sex	Age	Code	Source
M	27	D.E.	Wever, 1979 — Fig. 59

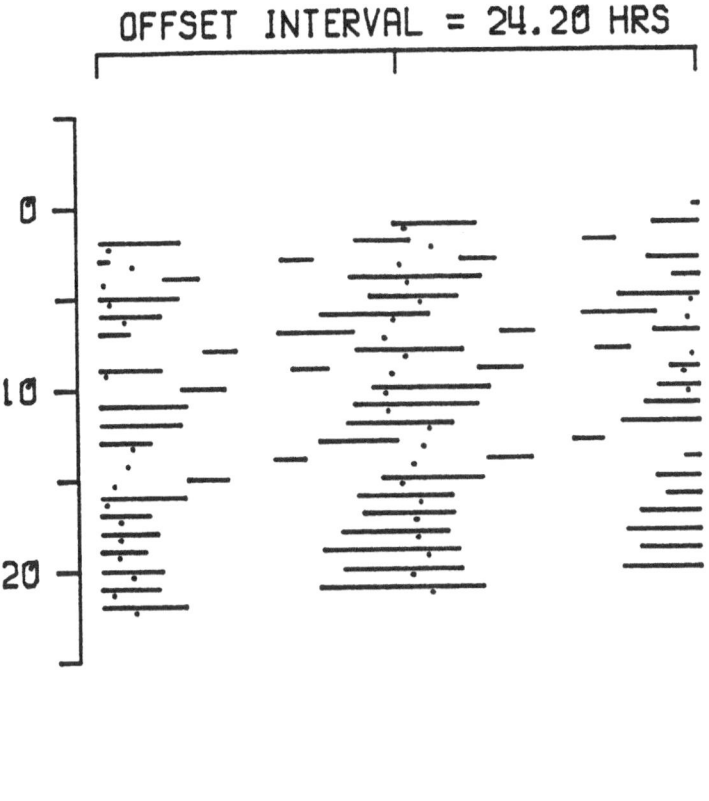

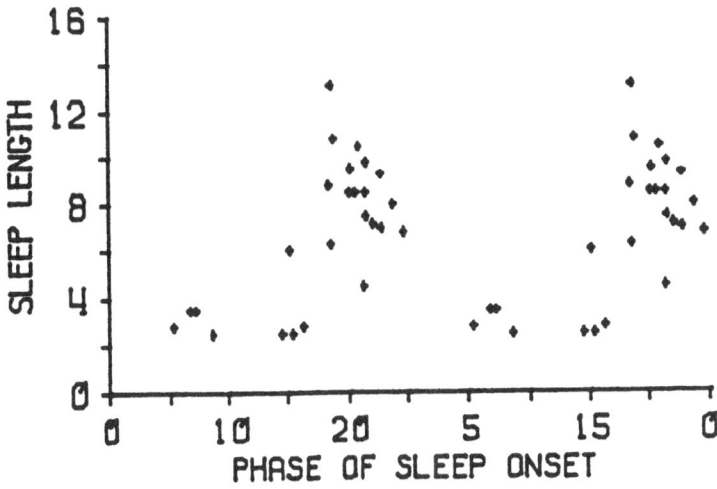

Figure 3-32. Normalized raster and sleep duration data for Subject 3.22.

Chapter 4

Patterns

Chapter 3 may have given the impression that sleep-wake records are highly variable. Indeed they are. Yet there are certain regularities or "patterns" which transcend the idiosyncrasies of individual subjects. Regarded in this way, each record becomes a variation on common themes.

To reveal some of these underlying patterns, I have re-analyzed sleep-wake and temperature data from long-term studies carried out by research groups in France, the United Kingdom, the United States and West Germany.

Subjects

The pooled data analyzed in Sections 4.1-4.6 were drawn from the first 15 subjects of Chapter 3, all of whom exhibited spontaneous internal desynchronization with a lengthening of the sleep-wake cycle. The 15 human subjects considered here were isolated from time cues for a combined total of more than two years, during which time 355 sleep episodes were recorded under conditions of spontaneous internal desynchronization.

Data Analysis

Sleep-wake records were normalized in the manner described at the beginning of Chapter 3 (Figure 3-2). Then for each sleep-wake cycle in each record, the following parameters were calculated: the lengths of sleep and wake episodes; the wake-sleep cycle length; and the circadian phases of sleep onset and wake-up. These data were pooled across subjects and then computer graphics were used to search for relationships among the various sleep-wake parameters.

Overview of Chapter 4

The first six sections address empirical relationships involving the duration of self-selected sleep and wake episodes, and their timing relative to the circadian cycle of body temperature. Even more than in Chapter 3, the emphasis is on free-running, internally desynchronized subjects. The patterns extracted in these sections have implications for theories of sleep regulation, the effects of irregular work-rest schedules, and the treatment of certain insomnias. Sections 4.7 and 4.8 reconsider two patterns which have figured prominently in previous theoretical controversies. Section 4.9 mentions some isolated patterns, as well as others which have been sought but not yet detected — their absence is significant and in contradiction to some existing models of the sleep-wake cycle. Section 4.10 discusses a different body of data, drawn from free-running nappers and split sleepers. The chapter closes with a summary of the known patterns.

4.1 Durations Vary with Circadian Phase of Sleep Onset

4.1.1 Sleep Length

Czeisler (1978; Czeisler et al., 1980a) and Zulley et al. (1981, 1982) noticed an intriguing pattern in the length of sleep episodes recorded during desynchronized free-run. Although in desynchrony the sleep-wake rhythm ostensibly "breaks loose" from the temperature rhythm, the circadian oscillator controlling temperature exerts a strong and unexpected influence on sleep. In particular the length of a sleep episode depends on when sleep begins in the circadian cycle.

Our data confirm and extend these previous reports of a relationship between sleep length ρ and the circadian phase ϕ_s of sleep onset (Figure 4-1a). Sleep length descends from about 18h to 7h along a ramp-shaped curve, then jumps to 18h at a phase about 8-9h after mid-low temperature. Near this phase, sleep length is bimodal.

The method of least squares was used to fit a quadratic function, denoted $\hat{\rho}(\phi_s)$, to the raw data. This fitted curve may be regarded as an estimate of the average sleep length obtained at each circadian phase of sleep onset.

One technical point about the curve fitting procedure: the upper and lower parts of the ramp-shaped data cloud overlap near $\phi_s \sim 8 - 12$. To emphasize this ramp structure, the points in the lower section (arbitrarily defined by $\rho < 11.5$h) were replotted one cycle later, at $\phi_s \sim 33-37$, before the quadratic was fit to the data.

4.1.2 Prior Wake Length

The phase of sleep onset is also consistently related to the length of the prior wake episode (Figure 4-1b). In this case, the fitted quadratic function is denoted $\hat{\alpha}(\phi_s)$, the average prior wake length at each phase of sleep onset. Prior wake length increases with phase of sleep onset, whereas sleep length decreases (Figure 4-1a). Thus $\hat{\rho}(\phi_s)$ and $\hat{\alpha}(\phi_s)$ vary inversely as functions of circadian phase. The longest and shortest wakes (Figure 4-1b) overlap near $\phi_s = 18-23$, a reminder that there is also a phase where sleep length is bimodal (Figure 4-1a). Curiously, where one curve is bimodal the other is smooth. The jumps in both sets of data reflect the fact that almost no wake-ups occur (Winfree, 1983) on the falling part of the temperature cycle between $\phi = 18$ and $\phi = 0$ (see Section 4.3).

4.1.3 Wake-Sleep Cycle Length

The phase of sleep onset determines the lengths of *both* parts of the wake-sleep cycle, and hence determines their sum: the combined wake-sleep cycle length (Figure 4-1c). The square wave shape is remarkable for biological data. Its plateaus emphasize the constancy of cycle length observed in each of two regimes (denoted LONG and SHORT). The regimes are distinguished by circadian phase: roughly speaking, SHORT or LONG correspond to bedtimes when temperature is low or high, respectively. The total distribution of sleep onsets is bimodal (Figure 4-1d), although in each regime separately it is unimodal. (See Section 4.4 for discussion of the distribution of sleep onsets.)

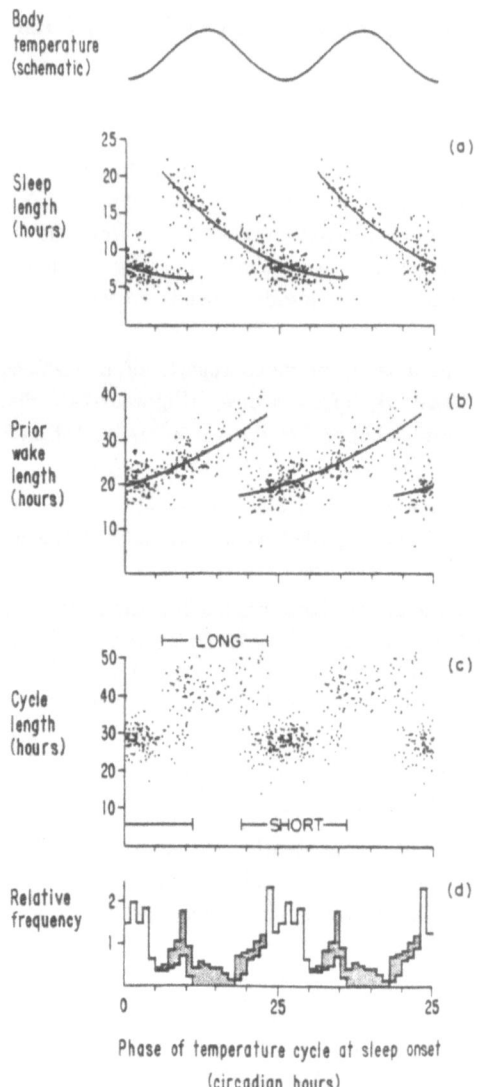

Figure 4-1

Circadian phase of sleep onset ϕ_s determines **(a)** subsequent sleep length ρ,
(b) prior wake length α, and **(c)** wake-sleep cycle length, defined as $\alpha + \rho$.
The method of least squares was used to fit quadratic functions $\hat{\rho}(\phi_s)$ and
$\hat{\alpha}(\phi_s)$ to the data of (a) and (b), respectively. The circadian cycle is divided
into 25 "circadian hours", with phase 0 at the mid-trough of the averaged
temperature rhythm. Note that data are double-plotted. **(d)** Histogram
showing the number of bedtimes selected at different circadian phases. The
vertical scale has been normalized so that a value of 1 corresponds to the
average frequency across all phases. The overall distribution is partitioned
into contributions from LONG (shaded) and SHORT.

4.1.4 Discussion

The dependence of sleep length on the circadian phase of bedtime (Figure 4-1a) has been reported by others (Czeisler, 1978; Czeisler *et al.*, 1980a; Zulley *et al.*, 1981, 1982) although they considered fewer sleep episodes (206 vs. 355 reported here). These sleep duration data have become a benchmark for the testing of models (Kronauer *et al.*, 1982; Daan *et al.*, 1984; Kawato *et al.*, 1982; Moore-Ede and Czeisler, 1984), first because the ϕ_s: ρ relationship is so clear, and second, because few alternative tests have been available.

The sleep length results have implications for the effects of irregular work schedules. Both in field studies of train drivers (Foret and Lantin, 1972) and in laboratory studies of normal subjects (Akerstedt and Gillberg, 1981) it has been demonstrated that sleeps were shortened as bedtime was delayed. After still longer wake extensions (Akerstedt and Gillberg, 1981) sleep lengthened abruptly, then declined again, similar to the shape of the ϕ_s: ρ relation in desynchronized free-run (Figure 4-1a). Thus, the shortened day-sleep of shift workers may be due not only to such disturbances as daytime noise, but also to the occurrence of bedtime relatively late in the circadian cycle.

To the best of my knowledge, Figure 4-1b depicts a new relationship. The quantitative relation between wake length and the circadian phase of the subsequent sleep onset is somewhat odd, since it is backwards in time; circadian phase of bedtime *retrodicts* the length of the prior wake episode. Others have sought a predictive relationship, e.g. wake length vs. phase of the temperature cycle at wake-up (Winfree, 1983; Zulley and Campbell, 1985) with varying success (Section 4.9.3). The main problem with using phase of wake-up as the independent variable is that it omits several hours of the circadian cycle — very few awakenings occur in the quarter-cycle before the temperature minimum (Section 4.3). All of the figures in this Section 4.1 would look far less structured if plotted relative to circadian phase of wake-up instead of phase of bedtime.

The finding of the square-wave relationship of Figure 4-1c is unexpected. Zulley (1983, 1985) has found (independently) a clustering of wake-sleep cycle lengths near 28h and 44h, a result now seen to follow from the dependence of cycle length on the circadian phase of bedtime.

4.2 Sleep Length and Prior Wake Length

4.2.1 α:ρ Scatterplot and Average Dependence on Circadian Phase

Figures 4-1a,b demonstrate that both sleep length and prior wake length are functions of circadian phase. How do sleep and prior wake length co-vary? A scatterplot of the raw data of ρ vs. α is shown in Figure 4-2. The main impression is that the data are noisy. Others (Winfree, 1982c) have commented on the apparent lack of structure in such scatterplots of sleep length vs. duration of prior wakefulness. A few features are clear: the data segregate into two diagonally sloping clouds, in each of which α and ρ are negatively correlated. The two clouds correspond point by point to the SHORT and LONG regimes noted earlier (Figure 4-1c).

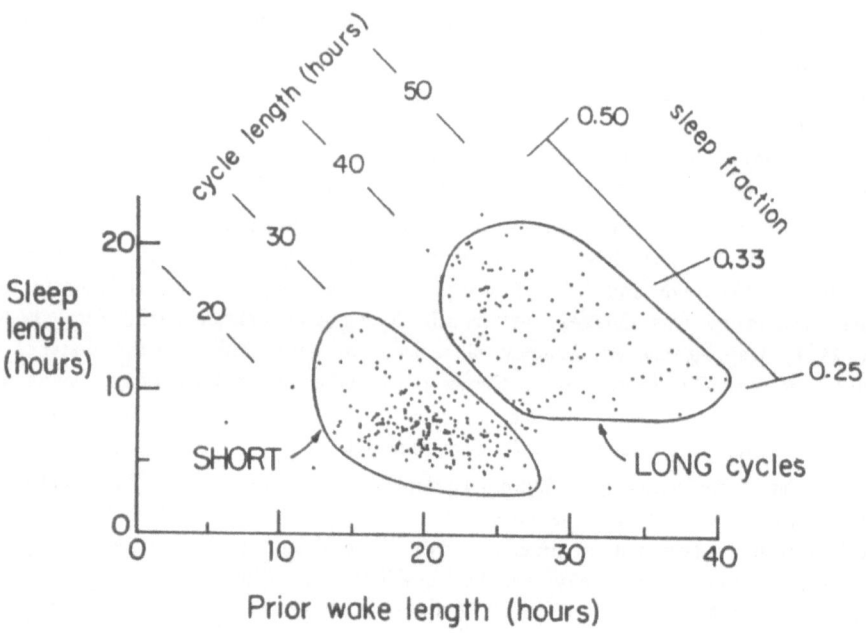

Figure 4-2. Scatterplot of sleep length vs. length of the prior wake episode. The data segregate into two diagonal clouds, corresponding to LONG and SHORT wake-sleep cycles as in Figure 4-1c. Cycle length and sleep fraction vary widely within each cloud.

It is possible to clarify Figure 4-2 by incorporating circadian phase information and by averaging out some of the scatter in the raw data. To this end we use the fitted curves $\hat{\rho}(\phi_s)$ and $\hat{\alpha}(\phi_s)$ of Figures 4-1a,b. The strategy is as follows: rather than plotting the raw α:ρ data, we plot instead the average values $\hat{\alpha}(\phi_s)$ and $\hat{\rho}(\phi_s)$ as ϕ_s moves through the circadian cycle. The joint variation of $\hat{\alpha}$ and $\hat{\rho}$ is shown in Figure 4-3. Axes derived from Figures 4-1a,b show the variation of circadian phase ϕ_s along the curves.

The construction of Figure 4-3 is based on a repetitive sequence of steps: (i) Select a circadian phase (ϕ_s) of sleep onset. (ii) Refer to Figure 4-1a and determine the average sleep length $\hat{\rho}(\phi_s)$ at that circadian phase. (iii) From Figure 4-1b determine the average length of prior wakefulness $\hat{\alpha}(\phi_s)$. (iv) Plot $\hat{\rho}$ vs. $\hat{\alpha}$. (v) Return to step (i), and choose a new phase. Steps (i)-(v) are repeated until the entire circadian cycle has been covered.

For example, at $\phi_s = 0$ we see from Figure 4-1a that $\hat{\rho}(0) = 8.1$h and from Figure 4-1b that $\hat{\alpha}(0) = 19.7$h. Therefore the point $(\hat{\alpha},\hat{\rho}) = (19.7, 8.1)$ is plotted on Figure 4-3. At that point on the curve, the adjacent tick mark with the 0 attached shows that the relevant phase of sleep onset is $\phi_s = 0$. As a second example, at $\phi_s = 10$, $\hat{\rho}$ has *two* values, one long (16.9h) and one short (6.3h), while $\hat{\alpha}$ has the single value $\hat{\alpha}(10) = 25.0$h (Figure 4-1a,b). Therefore for $\phi_s = 10$ we plot *two* points on Figure 4-3: one at $(\hat{\alpha},\hat{\rho}) = (25.0, 6.3)$ and one at $(\hat{\alpha},\hat{\rho}) = (25.0, 16.9)$. Each has a tick mark with $\phi_s = 10$ attached. Proceeding in this way for other ϕ_s, we complete the curves in Figure 4-3.

The shading along the curve indicates the number of sleep onsets which occur in each 1h bin of circadian phase. The bin populations are divided into three equal groups, with black, grey, or white bins in order of decreasing population. As shown in Figure 4-1d, the most likely phases of sleep onset are near $\phi = 0$ (mid-low temperature) and $\phi = 10$h later. Therefore the bins corresponding to those phases have been blackened in Figure 4-3.

Figure 4-3 summarizes a great deal of information. Unlike Figure 4-2, it includes circadian phase, as indicated by the derived phase axes running along the two branches of the curve. Figure 4-3 also shows how the density of sleep onsets varies with the phase of bedtime. Most importantly it elucidates the α:ρ relationship during internal desynchronization — the average relationship is a two-branched curve. On each branch α and ρ are negatively correlated. Moreover the branches are distinguished by the circadian phase of sleep onset. Wake-sleep cycle length is approximately constant on each branch (averaging 28h and 42h, respectively), whereas daily sleep fraction varies considerably on each branch.

4.2.2 Uncorrelated residuals of α and ρ

Thus far we have emphasized the circadian variation of sleep length and prior wake length. In particular, the construction of Figure 4-3 depended on studying the average circadian components $\hat{\rho}(\phi_s)$ and $\hat{\alpha}(\phi_s)$ in Figures 4-1a,b; we have neglected any discussion of the residual deviations of the observed data about those fitted curves. These residuals may contain interesting information.

By considering the residuals of α and ρ about their fitted curves, we may test a simple restorative model for the control of sleep duration. This model is motivated by a question about the scatter in Figures 4-1a,b: at a fixed phase ϕ_s of sleep onset, why are some sleep episodes longer than others? Any explanation based on circadian phase is ruled out,

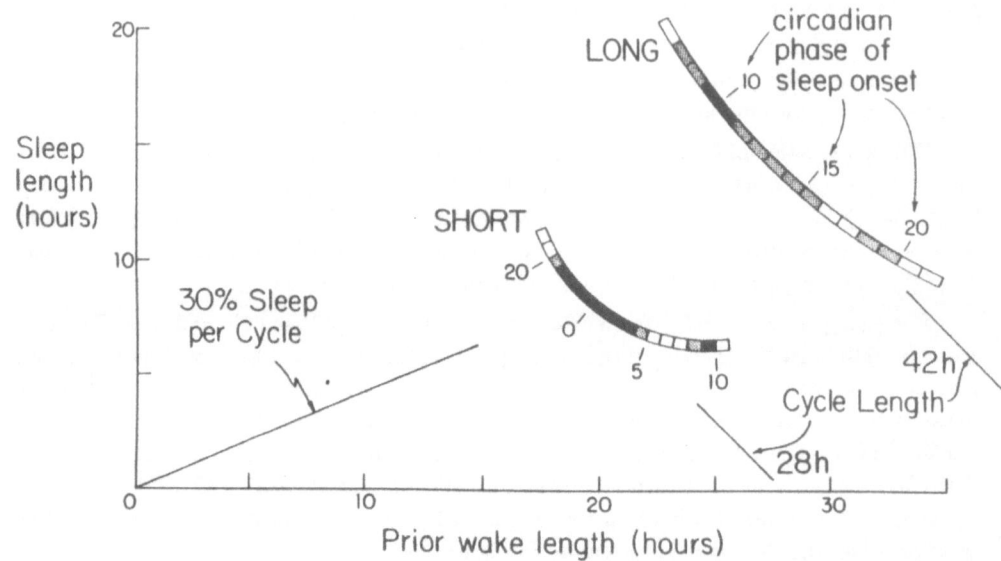

Figure 4-3. Covariations of average sleep and prior wake length, conditioned on phase of sleep onset. The average curves in Figures 4-1a,b are here replotted to reveal their joint variation. The circadian cycle is divided into 25 bins, each about 1h wide: bin 0 begins at phase 0, the mid-trough of the temperature rhythm. Circadian phases of sleep onset are numbered along the curves. The phase bins have been divided into three equal groups and shaded such that darker sections of the curve represent more frequently selected phases of bedtime. The cycle lengths of SHORT and LONG are about 28h and 42h, respectively. Daily sleep fraction averages about 0.3, but is highly variable. In both SHORT and LONG, sleep length and prior wake length vary inversely.

because ϕ_s is being controlled for, i.e., the phase of bedtime is the same for the sleep episodes in question. The restorative model tries to relate the differences in sleep length to differences in the length of prior wakefulness. It claims that, given two sleep episodes beginning at phase ϕ_s, the longer sleep episode will be that preceded by the longer wake episode.

In other words, after correcting for the dependence on circadian phase, any further lengthening of sleep might be due to an unusually long and tiring bout of prior wakefulness. This expectation would follow from a restorative model for sleep duration. To test it, we have calculated the deviations of sleep and wake length from the fitted curves of Figures 4-1a,b. As shown in Figure 4-4 we find no significant positive correlation between these deviations $(r = -0.10)$, contrary to the prediction of the restorative model. Thus, circadian phase of sleep onset determines the average lengths of subsequent sleep and prior wake; above and beyond their phase-mediated relationship, these lengths are uncorrelated.

To avoid possible confusion, we stress that it is the *residuals* which are uncorrelated. More formally, the residuals $\Delta\rho$ and $\Delta\alpha$ for each episode are defined by

$$\Delta\rho \;=\; \rho - \hat{\rho}(\phi_s)$$

$$\Delta\alpha \;=\; \alpha - \hat{\alpha}(\phi_s) \,.$$

The novel aspect of this calculation is that we have corrected for the average circadian components $\hat{\alpha}(\phi_s)$ and $\hat{\rho}(\phi_s)$ of α and ρ, respectively. The more usual calculation (Aschoff et al., 1971; Wever, 1979, 1984a) concerns the correlation of the raw data, α and ρ, *without* prior removal of the circadian components. When adjustment is made for such circadian variations, the residuals $\Delta\alpha$ and $\Delta\rho$ are not significantly correlated. This lack of correlation is a damaging blow to the restorative model discussed above.

4.2.3 Discussion

$\alpha{:}\rho$ Relationship During Synchrony and Desynchrony

We have found that the average $\alpha{:}\rho$ relationship during internal desynchronization is a two-branched curve (Figure 4-3) with branches distinguished by circadian phase. On each of these branches, α and ρ are negatively correlated. ($r = -0.47$ on the SHORT branch, and $r = -0.43$ on the LONG branch.) As will now be discussed, these results unify and reconcile earlier work on $\alpha{:}\rho$ correlations for internally synchronized (Aschoff et al., 1971; Wever, 1979; 1984a) and desynchronized (Czeisler et al., 1980a) subjects.

Several authors have studied the lengths of the self-selected sleep episodes observed during free-run. For internally synchronized subjects, sleep length (ρ) was found to be negatively correlated $(r = -0.53 \pm 0.22)$ to length of prior wakefulness (α) (Wever, 1984a). However, for internally desynchronized subjects, Czeisler et al. (1980a) reported a positive serial correlation $(r = +0.41)$ between α and ρ.

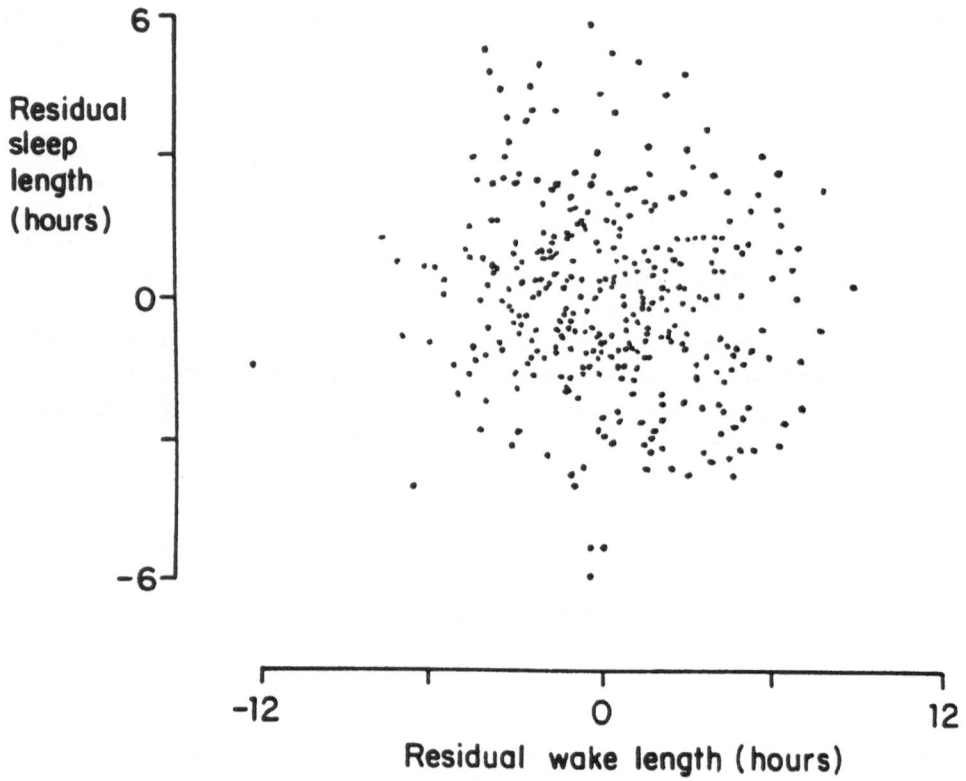

Figure 4-4. Bivariate distribution of residuals of sleep length and prior wake length. Residuals are defined as deviations from the circadian phase-adjusted mean curves of Figures 4-1a,b. Note that the axes are drawn to different scales to reflect the relative proportions of sleep and wake in the sleep-wake cycle. There is no significant positive correlation among the residuals, contrary to the prediction of restorative models.

Why is the $\alpha{:}\rho$ correlation negative during synchrony and positive during desynchrony? It turns out that a correlation coefficient is inadequate to capture the subtle structure of the $\alpha{:}\rho$ relationship during desynchrony. The main defect of the correlation coefficient is that it ignores circadian phase. By lumping episodes together independent of their timing in the circadian cycle, vital information is lost. By taking circadian phase into account, we now show that the desynchronized $\alpha{:}\rho$ relationship is fully compatible with and indeed subsumes the synchronized case.

Synchronized subjects sample only the lower branch (SHORT) of Figure 4-3, because they invariably fall asleep near the trough of the body temperature cycle (by definition of internal synchrony). Note that on the SHORT branch of the $\alpha{:}\rho$ relationship (Figures 4-2, 4-3) α and ρ are clearly negatively correlated. Indeed if we calculate the $\alpha{:}\rho$ correlation for only the SHORT cloud in Figure 4-2, we obtain $r = -0.47$, which agrees with the result $r = -0.53 \pm 0.22$ obtained for internally synchronized subjects (Wever, 1984a). This finding suggests that synchronized and desynchronized subjects do not differ in their intrinsic $\alpha{:}\rho$ control mechanisms: they differ in that desynchronized subjects occasionally sample the LONG branch whereas synchronized subjects never do.

Furthermore, Figure 4-3 accounts for the positive $\alpha{:}\rho$ correlation observed in desynchronized subjects. These subjects most often sample the SHORT and LONG branches near $\phi = 0$ and $\phi = 10$, respectively. These are the blackened bins in Figure 4-3. Note that these bins lie along a diagonal line of *positive* slope. Since they are most heavily populated, the dark bins dominate the correlation calculation, leading to a positive $\alpha{:}\rho$ correlation for desynchronized subjects. The value we obtain for the $\alpha{:}\rho$ correlation during desynchrony is $r = 0.34$, close to the value of $r = 0.41$ reported for a smaller sample (Czeisler et al., 1980a).

Uncorrelated Residuals of α and ρ:
Implications for Restorative Models of Sleep Duration

The surprising finding of Section 4.2.2 concerns the residual deviations of α and ρ from their circadian phase-adjusted mean values: The residuals show no significant positive cross-correlation. This result contradicts a restorative model for the control of sleep duration.

Animal studies have been conducted to address restorative models. Webb and Friedmann (1969) found no relationship between sleep and wake lengths in rats on a 12:12 light-dark schedule. On the other hand, Mistlberger et al. (1984) studied suprachiasmatic nuclei (SCN) lesioned rats free-running in constant dim light, thereby attenuating the circadian regulation of sleep and wake. They reported significant positive correlations between the lengths of successive sleep and wake episodes. In particular, sleep was claimed to be not only restorative but also "preparative"; very long sleeps were likely to be followed by very long wakes. Taken together, the studies suggest that circadian regulation normally dominates any homeostatic control of sleep duration. In rats, homeostasis is only revealed by SCN lesions; in intact humans, homeostatic influences on spontaneous sleep duration are weak or absent.

In assessing the theoretical consequences of the results of Section 4.2.2, it is important to distinguish between two possible restorative models. The first and simplest asserts that the length of an unrestricted sleep episode increases with the length of prior wakefulness. This model was refuted long ago by studies (Aschoff *et al.*, 1971) of free-running humans with internally synchronized circadian rhythms, in which a negative $\alpha{:}\rho$ correlation was observed. A second, more sophisticated restorative model claims that the negative $\alpha{:}\rho$ correlation merely reflects the dominance of circadian regulation: if the circadian influence could be eliminated somehow, then (according to this second model) the homeostatic control of sleep duration would become evident. As mentioned above, Mistlberger *et al.* (1984) followed the strategy of experimentally eliminating circadian influences, and their results were consistent with this second restorative model. The present study introduces a test of the second model as applied to free-running humans. Statistics rather than surgery were used to remove circadian influences on sleep duration. The finding is that, after correction is made for the circadian-mediated correlation of α and ρ, the residual lengths $\Delta\alpha$ and $\Delta\rho$ of sleep and prior wake are *uncorrelated*, in contradiction to the second restorative model. Homeostatic mechanisms serve mainly to regulate the amount of slow-wave sleep (Borbely, 1982) rather than the overall duration of sleep. Apparently it is the circadian system, not the prior sleep-wake history, which is most important in governing the length of unrestricted wake and sleep in man.

4.3 Timing of Wake-Up

During 24h-entrainment or free-running internal synchrony, sleep is confined to one part of the circadian temperature cycle. But during internal desynchrony, the sleep-wake cycle moves in and out of phase with the temperature rhythm. This section and the next two address the timing of sleep and wake in relation to the phase of the circadian clock. For example, are desynchronized subjects equally likely to fall asleep at any circadian phase, or are some phases preferred? On the other hand, is there an "internal alarm clock" which wakes the subjects at a precise phase? This latter question will be discussed now.

The simplest approach is to plot the distribution of the observed phases of wake-up. I have divided the circadian cycle into 25 bins, each about 1h wide; bin 0 begins at phase $\phi = 0$, the mid-trough of the average temperature rhythm.

Wake-up nearly always occurs when temperature is rising (Figure 4-5). In the first half of the cycle, 85% of the wake-ups occur. (Based on a sample one-third the size of that studied here, Czeisler *et al.* (1980a) reported a similar value of 86%).

Note however that the histogram is broad. Apparently the internal alarm clock doesn't ring at the same time in each cycle. More precisely, wake-up is timed by sleep onset according to a curvilinear relationship, as we have seen in Figure 4-1. If the curve of Figure 4-1a were a line of slope $= -1$, all sleep episodes would end at the same phase. Since the observed slope is always less negative than -1, later sleep onsets lead to (slightly) later wake-up.

There is a "sleep-maintenance zone" near $\phi = 17{-}25$. Sleeping subjects tend to maintain their sleep through this zone where body temperature is below its mean and falling. As Winfree (1983) has emphasized, the zone of forbidden wake-up is mathematically equivalent to the gap between long and short sleeps occurring near $\phi_s = 8$ in the $\phi_s{:}\rho$ data of Figure 4-1a.

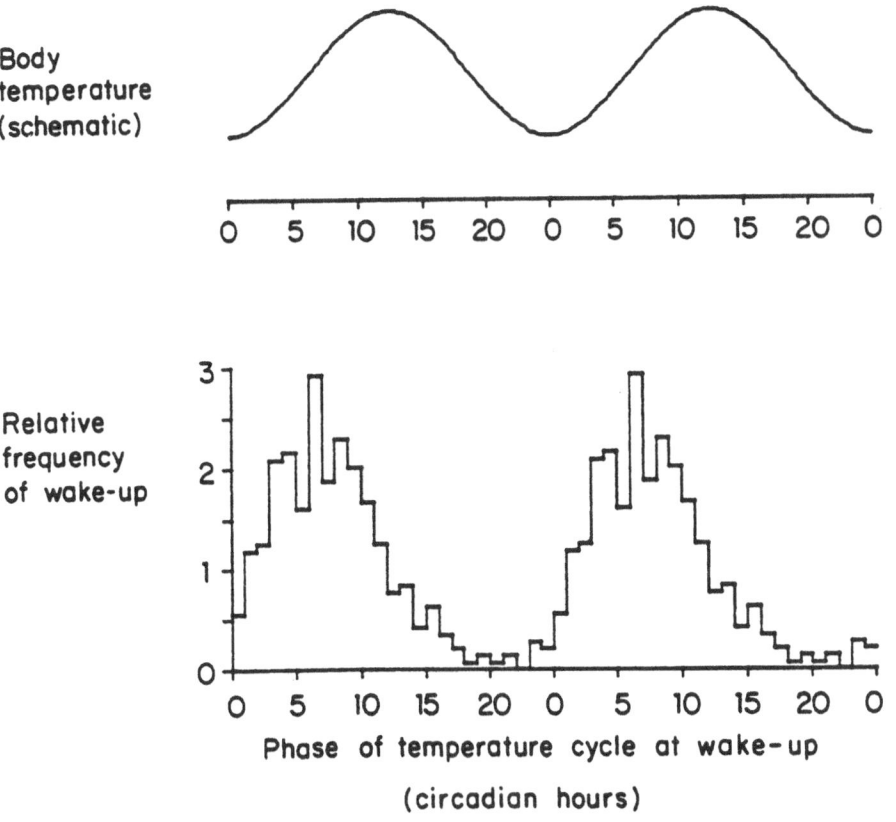

Distribution of spontaneous awakenings during
internally desynchronized free-run (N =15 subjects)

Body
temperature
(schematic)

0   5   10   15   20   0   5   10   15   20   0

Relative
frequency
of wake-up

3

2

1

0

0   5   10   15   20   0   5   10   15   20   0

Phase of temperature cycle at wake-up

(circadian hours)

Figure 4-5. Distribution of wake-ups during internal desynchronization. The
vertical scale is normalized such that a relative frequency of 1 corresponds to
the mean value across all phases. Most awakenings occur on the rising limb
of the temperature cycle.

The zone of forbidden wake-up is important for several reasons: (1) Rotating shift workers or airplane pilots may be forced to get up at this time — what are the consequences for their health and performance? This question deserves experimental study. (2) The zone strongly constrains the shape of the relation between phase of sleep onset, prior wake length and sleep length (Figures 4-1a,b) by producing diagonal channels from which data are practically absent. These channels are just redescriptions, graphical echoes of the zone (Figure 4-6), and not new phenomena requiring biological explanation. In this way the jumps of Figures 4-1a and 4-1b are linked. (However, the zone of forbidden wake-up does *not* explain why the jumps occur at the phases that they do — that requires a second process, one governing sleep onset.)

4.4 Timing of Sleep Onset

4.4.1 Histograms from Internally Desynchronized Subjects in Free-Run

The analysis of Section 4.3 is now applied to sleep onset, rather than wake-up. In contrast to the unimodal distribution of awakenings, the histogram of sleep onsets has two peaks in the circadian cycle (Figure 4-7). The major peak near $\phi = 0$ corresponds to a lethargic phase observed in other studies: subjective alertness (Czeisler *et al.*, 1980a) and performance on various tasks (Colquhoun, 1972) are lowest then, while propensity for REM sleep is highest (Czeisler *et al.*, 1980a,b).

The second peak ($\phi = 9{-}10$) is a novel result. It corresponds to the "mid-day dip" (Richardson *et al.*, 1982) observed in subjects entrained to a 24h day. (Taking 6-7 AM as a typical time of low temperature in young entrained subjects (Czeisler *et al.*, 1986) indicates that $\phi = 9$ corresponds to 3-4 PM, i.e. siesta time). Others (Webb, 1978a; Broughton, 1975, 1983) have speculated that our endogenous rhythm of sleep tendency is bimodal and hence that afternoon napping is biologically, as well as culturally, based. Figure 4-7 is to my knowledge the first report of a peak at nap phase in free-running internally desynchronized humans.

Nevertheless the peak at $\phi = 9$ is not due to naps in the usual sense; the sleep episodes begin after about 25h of prior wake (Figure 4-1b) and may last for over 20h (Figure 4-1a). Most of the free-running subjects studied here were instructed to "sleep only when tired" and to "avoid naps". Without this injunction, true naps might have been observed more often (cf. Zulley and Campbell, 1985).

Zulley *et al.* (1981, 1982) have also reported a bimodal distribution of sleep onsets. Their sample is smaller (206 episodes vs. 355 reported here) and their reported phases disagree with ours, probably because their reference phase is the cycle-by-cycle observed temperature minimum, a measure heavily contaminated by the masking effects of sleep, exercise, posture, showers, etc.

The rhythm of sleep tendency may even be multimodal (Kronauer *et al.*, 1985). By pooling records, one can inadvertently smear delicate peaks. Certainly some subjects (Sections 3.7, 3.9) tantalize us with 3 or 4 sharp peaks, hinting at ultradian substructure on a 6-8h time scale.

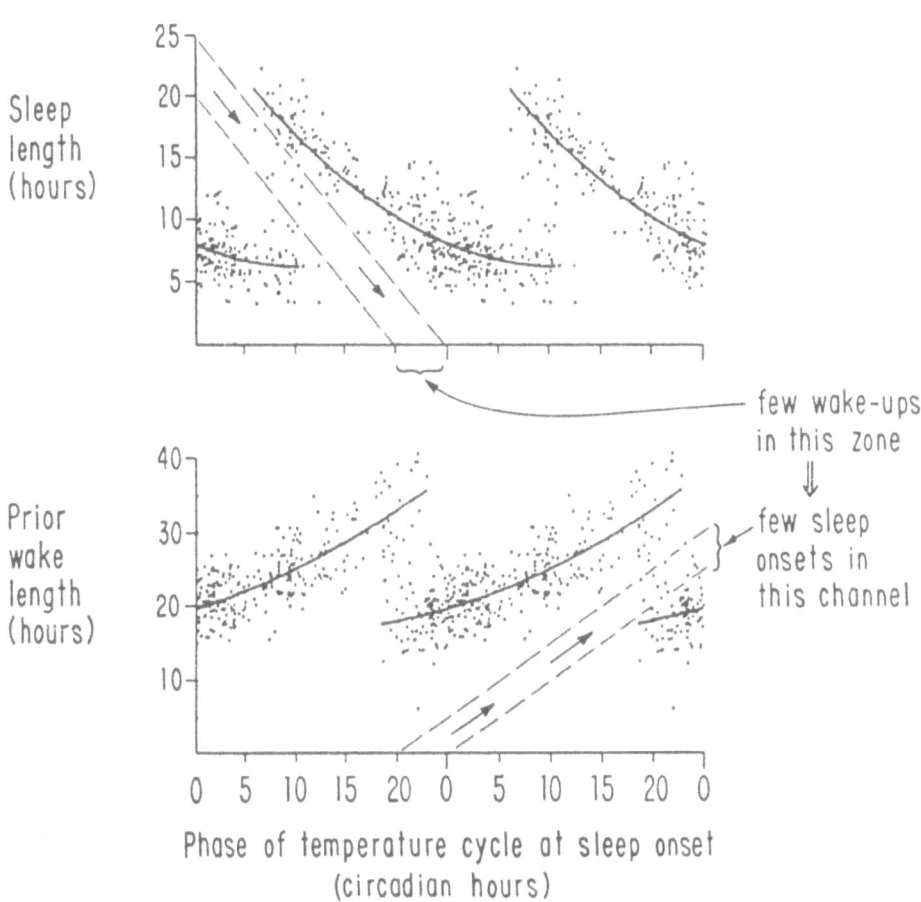

Jumps in sleep length
and in prior wake length:
Relation to zone of forbidden
wake-up

Sleep length (hours)

Prior wake length (hours)

few wake-ups
in this zone
⇓
few sleep
onsets in
this channel

Phase of temperature cycle at sleep onset
(circadian hours)

Figure 4-6.

(**Top**): On the $\phi_s{:}\rho$ plane, circadian phase of wake-up is constant along lines of slope $= -1$, since $\rho = \phi_w - \phi_s$. Hence the few data in the diagonal channel (dashed lines) are precisely those which give rise to awakenings between $\phi = 20$ and $\phi = 25 = 0$.

(**Bottom**): On the $\alpha{:}\phi_s$ plane, circadian phase of preceding wake-up is constant along lines of slope $= +1$, since $\alpha = \phi_s - \phi_w$. Because there are few wake episodes beginning in the zone of "forbidden" wake-up, there are (as a tautology) few data in the diagonal channel of slope $= +1$ (dashed lines) leading from that zone.

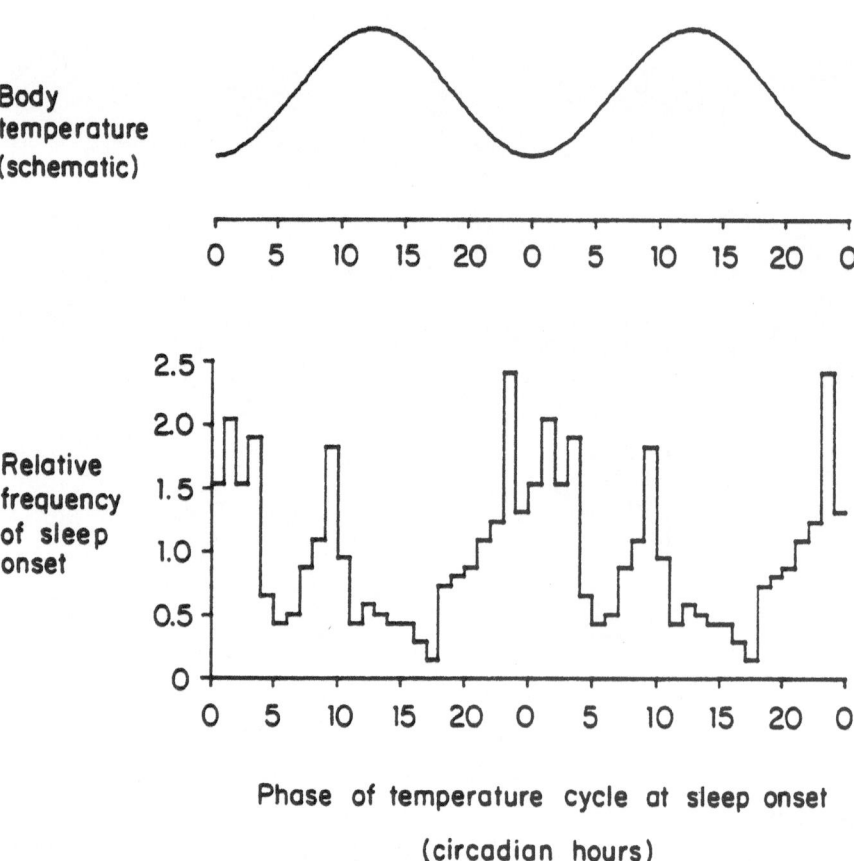

Bimodal distribution of self-selected
bedtimes during internally desynchronized
free-run (N = 15 subjects)

Body
temperature
(schematic)

Relative
frequency
of sleep
onset

Phase of temperature cycle at sleep onset

(circadian hours)

Figure 4-7. Distribution of self-selected bedtimes during internal desynchronization. The vertical scale is normalized such that a frequency of 1 corresponds
to the mean value across all phases. Compare Figures 4-1d and 4-12.

4.4.2 "BEDCHECK" and the Rate of Sleep Onset

The histograms of Section 4.4.1 beg the question: how much do such distributions reflect the underlying rhythm of sleep propensity? After all, the observed wake-up distribution is far from uniform (Section 4.3) — so perhaps certain potential bedtimes are favored simply because more subjects have been awake a long time when they get to those phases and are therefore sleepier at them. Other phases may have few sleep onsets because of a lack of opportunity — for example, subjects cannot fall asleep if they already *are* asleep. Likewise, they are unlikely to fall asleep if they have just awakened.

The aim of this section is to study the differential opportunities for sleep in the circadian cycle. Taking these data into account allows one to calculate a "rate of sleep onset" in which *opportunity* for sleep plays no part.

4.4.2.1 BEDCHECK

When are internally desynchronized subjects apt to be asleep? Figure 4-8 shows the percent of time the subjects are in bed, as a function of circadian phase. (I call this graph BEDCHECK, a term borrowed from the parlance of overnight summer-camp.) Few other graphs of sleep data are as sinusoidal as this one, which has a maximum of 52% near $\phi = 3$, a flat minimum of 23% near $\phi = 13-19$, and a mean value of 33%, which represents an overall average sleep fraction for the 15 subjects considered here. Not surprisingly, subjects are most likely to be in bed just after $\phi = 0$, the sleepy time marked by the temperature nadir. It is harder to say why $\phi \sim 13-19$ is physiologically special, but for some reason subjects are rarely asleep then. As will be shown in Section 4.5, several other sorts of measures indicate that $\phi \sim 16-19$ is, so to speak, an activated time in the circadian cycle.

4.4.2.2 Rate of Sleep Onset

To estimate the circadian variation of sleep tendency, it is important to tease out the relative contributions of circadian phase and prior wakefulness; both affect the timing of sleep onset. The trouble is that the two variables are not independent. As was seen in Figure 4-1b, longer wake episodes are associated with later circadian phases of sleep onset. On average, the longer a desynchronized free-running subject stays awake, the later in the cycle he will fall asleep. This is not a tautology, however, since it relies on the experimental fact that most wake episodes begin near a common phase, namely the rising slope of the temperature rhythm (Section 4.3).

Thus the observed sleep onset distribution (Figure 4-7) poses a problem of interpretation. For example, given that few sleep episodes begin at a particular circadian phase, is it merely because the subjects haven't been awake long enough to feel sleepy, or is it because the sleep tendency is genuinely low at that phase in the circadian cycle?

We need to find some way to control for "sleep opportunity" and prior wakefulness. One approach, devised by Richard Kronauer in response to some constructive criticism offered by Serge Daan and Domien Beersma, involves conditioning on the phase of wake-up. It is best illustrated by the following thought experiment.

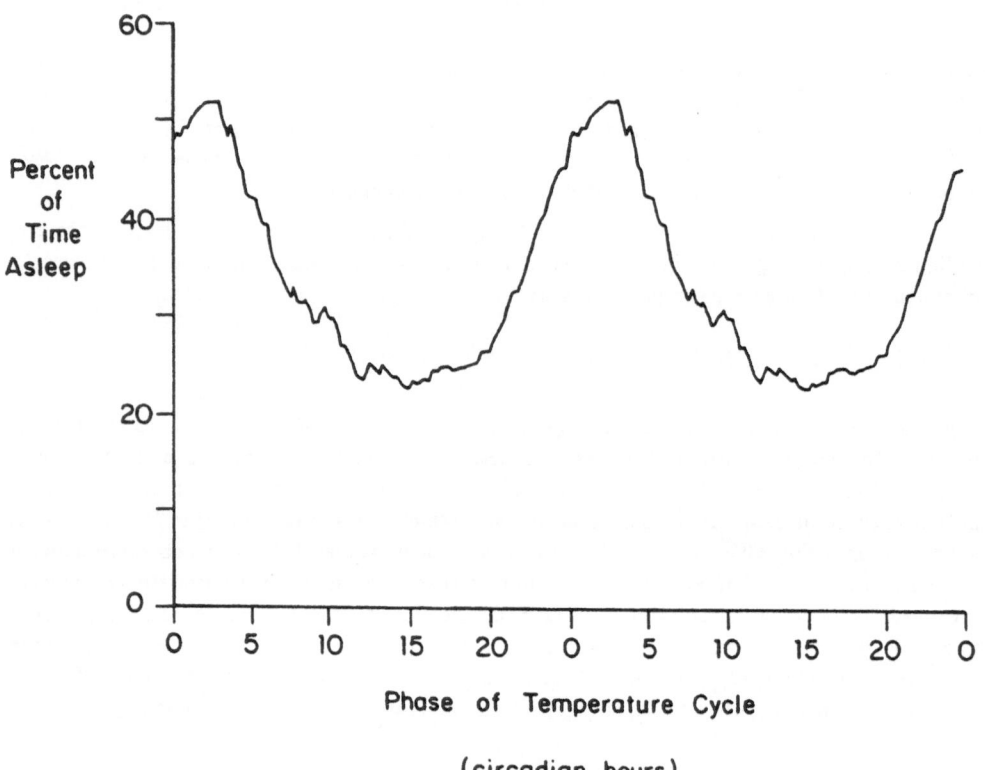

Figure 4-8. BEDCHECK: The percent of time that desynchronized subjects are found in bed at various phases of the circadian cycle. In the computation of the average, each subject's record (not each sleep episode) was given equal weight.

Cohorts

Consider a population of subjects who all happen to wake up at a certain phase, say phase $\phi = 5$ for definiteness. Call this collection of subjects a "cohort." As the members of this cohort get out bed, eat breakfast, and go through their free-running routine, two things are happening: wake length is increasing, and the subjects are passing through the circadian cycle (Figure 4-9). The cohort is marching through time and, like a population of radioactive atoms, every so often some of them will decay, i.e. fall asleep. As the cohort passes through very sleepy phases of the cycle, many of its members will fall asleep. Here "many" must mean on a *percentage* basis. (It is not fair to compare later phases to earlier ones in terms of *absolute* numbers of decays, since necessarily fewer subjects are available to later phases, some having decayed in the meantime.)

A rate of sleep onset can be calculated for the cohort, as a function of circadian phase. Divide the cycle into 25 bins, and let $N(\phi)$ be the number of subjects still awake in bin ϕ. Then $\Delta N = N(\phi) - N(\phi+1)$ is the number of subjects who have fallen asleep in the 1 hour bin ϕ. Hence $(\Delta N)/N$ is the fractional rate of decay, as a function of phase.

An example of such a rate curve is shown in Figure 4-10. Because there are only 355 desynchronized sleep episodes available from the data bank of Chapter 3, we resort to a coarse definition of cohort. Cohort #1 consists of all those wake episodes ($N = 119$) beginning between $\phi = 0$ and $\phi = 6$. The dashed curve shows that one cycle later, the maximal rate of sleep onset is about 30% per hour, near $\phi = 2$ and $\phi = 10$. In other words, about 30% of the surviving members of the cohort fall asleep in those 1 hour bins, which correspond to the sleep and nap phases identified earlier (Section 4.4.1). On the other hand, the rate is only about 7% per hour near $\phi = 6$. Subjects generally maintain their wakefulness through this zone (see Section 4.5 for a full discussion of wake-maintenance zones). The low rate cannot be ascribed to a lack of opportunity; there are still subjects awake in the cohort and indeed they march on to even later phases before falling asleep.

Now the calculation may be repeated for another cohort, say all those wakes ($N = 168$) beginning between $\phi = 6$ and $\phi = 12$ (Figure 4-10, solid curve). The beauty of this second calculation is that the rate curves for the two cohorts can be compared phase by phase. As they march through any given phase, the members of cohort #1 will have been awake about 6h longer than those in cohort #2, since they started the wake-episode about 6h earlier in the circadian cycle. *Thus the rate-enhancing effects of prolonged prior wakefulness can be cleanly assessed*, free from the confounding influence of varying circadian phase of sleep onset.

Analyzing the data in this manner reveals two striking features (Figure 4-10).

(1) The two rate curves nearly coincide over the interval $\phi = 5-12$, in spite of the additional six hours of wakefulness endured by cohort #1. Apparently the circadian component of sleep tendency dominates the prior wakefulness component. For example, at $\phi = 6$, cohort #1 has been awake about 27h, cohort #2 about 21h. All the same, both cohorts show a rate of sleep onset of 7% per hour.

(2) In the region of the temperature trough ($\phi \sim 0$), extra prior wakefulness makes a big difference. Cohort #1 nods off at a peak rate of 32% per hour, whereas Cohort #2 never exceeds 15%. The shape of the rate curves is similar, but #1 is always steeper. (On closer inspection, this steepness result holds for *all* phases. However, the effect is most pronounced

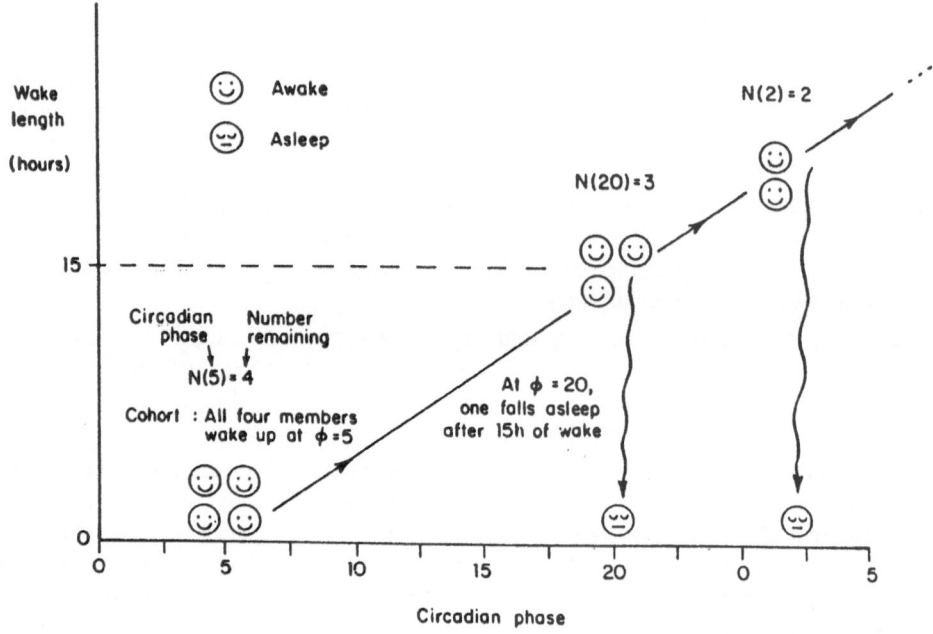

Figure 4-9. Explanation of "cohorts," a concept used in calculating the rate of sleep onset. A cohort consists of all those wake episodes (personified here as four cheery faces) which began at or near a particular circadian phase (here, $\phi = 5$). Transitions from wakefulness to sleep cause the relevant episodes to drop out of the cohort. The "survival function" $N(\phi)$ measures the number of wake episodes remaining in the cohort at phase ϕ. (Different cohorts would have different functions N.) See text and Figure 4-10 for the use of $N(\phi)$ in the calculation of the rate of sleep onset.

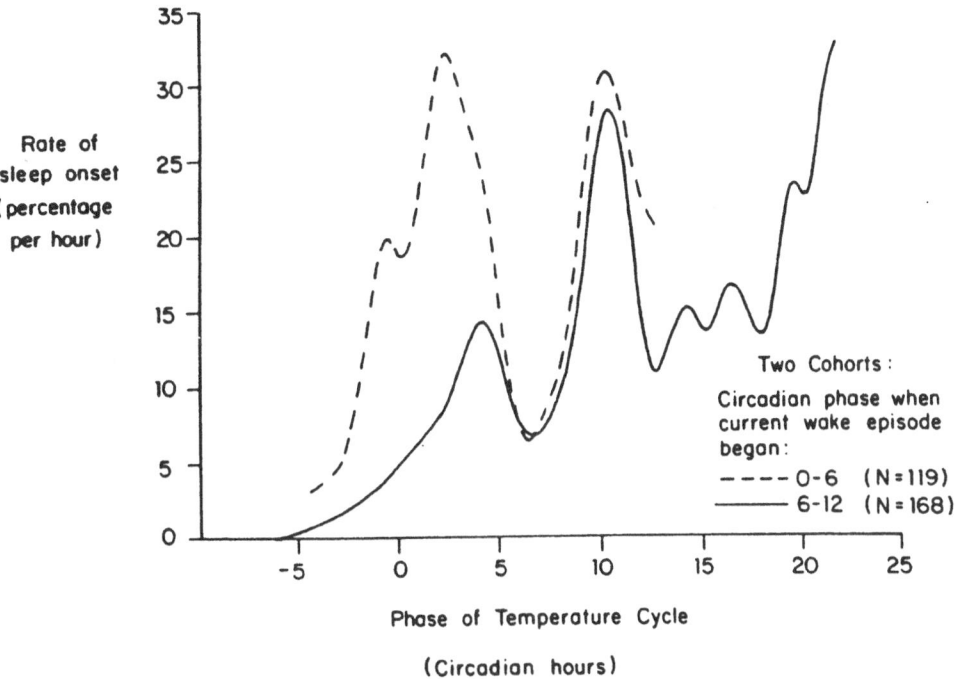

Percentage of subjects (currently awake at phase ϕ)
who fall asleep in the next hour

Rate of
sleep onset
(percentage
per hour)

Two Cohorts:

Circadian phase when
current wake episode
began:

- - - - 0-6 (N=119)
———— 6-12 (N=168)

Phase of Temperature Cycle

(Circadian hours)

Figure 4-10 Rate of sleep onset, as a function of circadian phase. The circadian cycle is divided into 25 bins. Rates are computed for cohort #1 (dashed line) consisting of 119 wake episodes beginning in $\phi \in [0,6]$ and for cohort #2 (solid line) consisting of 168 wake episodes beginning in $\phi \in [6,12]$. The circadian cycle shown is the next one after that in which the wake-up occurred.

The rates were computed in several steps: (1) Let $N(\phi)$ = number awake in bin ϕ. (2) The natural logarithm, $ln\ N(\phi)$ was plotted against ϕ. (3) The $ln\ N$ data were smoothed with a 3-point moving average (relative weights = 1,2,1). (4) The smoothed data were interpolated by a cubic spline. (5) The spline was differentiated, giving a smooth approximation

$$\frac{d}{d\phi}(ln\ N(\phi)) = \frac{dN}{d\phi}\frac{1}{N(\phi)} \sim \frac{\Delta N}{N}\frac{1}{\Delta\phi}$$

to the desired fractional rate of sleep onset.

I thank Andrew Ward for helping me with the spline.

at the temperature trough.)

These results suggest that prolonged wakefulness increases the *rate* of sleep onset, moreso at some phases than at others. The sleepiest time in the cycle — the temperature trough — appears particularly sensitive to the effects of prolonged wakefulness.

4.5 Wake-Maintenance Zones

In Section 4.3, we saw that spontaneous wake-up rarely occurs in the last quarter of the temperature cycle. Other evidence indicates that there are also zones in the cycle where sleep onsets are so rare as to be virtually forbidden. These zones are called "wake-maintenance zones", (Strogatz and Kronauer, 1985) because subjects who are awake tend to maintain their wakefulness through them. In what follows the zones will be defined more precisely, and they will be shown to be implicated in certain insomnias.

I wish to thank Richard Kronauer, who discovered and named the wake-maintenance zones, for allowing me to present several of his ideas here.

4.5.1 Zones in Free-Run

When sleep-wake records from internally desynchronized subjects are replotted in a normalized raster (Figure 3-2), they show a remarkable unity in the occurrence and placement of the wake-maintenance zones (Figure 4-11). Notice that in the four subjects shown in Figure 4-11, no black bars ever begin in the stippled zones. In other words, subjects avoided bedtime at those phases in the temperature cycle. The zones occur about 8h before, and about 6h after the temperature minimum. They are about 2-3h wide, and could be even wider in some of the cases shown. (The same minimal zones are drawn for all, to emphasize their universality across subjects.) The invariance of the zones is especially impressive when one recalls how different the subjects are in other ways: sleep fractions range from 0.30 to 0.36, and average sleep-wake cycles range from 29 to 40h.

When the sleep onset phases from 15 desynchronized subjects in the data bank (Chapter 3) are pooled, we obtain the histogram of sleep onsets shown in Figure 4-12 (cf. Figure 4-7, from Section 4.4.1). The wake-maintenance zones appear as local minima.

Figure 4-12 contains the first hint that the zones may be implicated in some insomnias. If we assume that these free-run data bear on 24h entrainment, then we can convert circadian phases to approximate times of day by noting that for college age students with a habitual waketime near 8:30 AM, the unmasked trough of temperature occurs near 6-7 AM (Czeisler, 1985; Czeisler *et al.*, 1986). This means that one zone (henceforth the "morning zone") occurs near 12 noon, and the other ("evening zone") occurs near 10 PM, just before entrained bedtime. With the evening zone normally perched so close to bedtime, we can imagine disorders in which — for some reason — sleep onset is actually attempted in the zone. Then sleep-onset insomnia could result, as it often seems to when we try to fall asleep an hour or two earlier than usual.

Is the evening zone implicated in sleep-onset insomnia? All that has been shown so far is that free-running subjects rarely fall asleep in the zones; but would they find it *difficult* to do so, were they to try? After all, that is the crux of sleep-onset insomnia: the wake-sleep

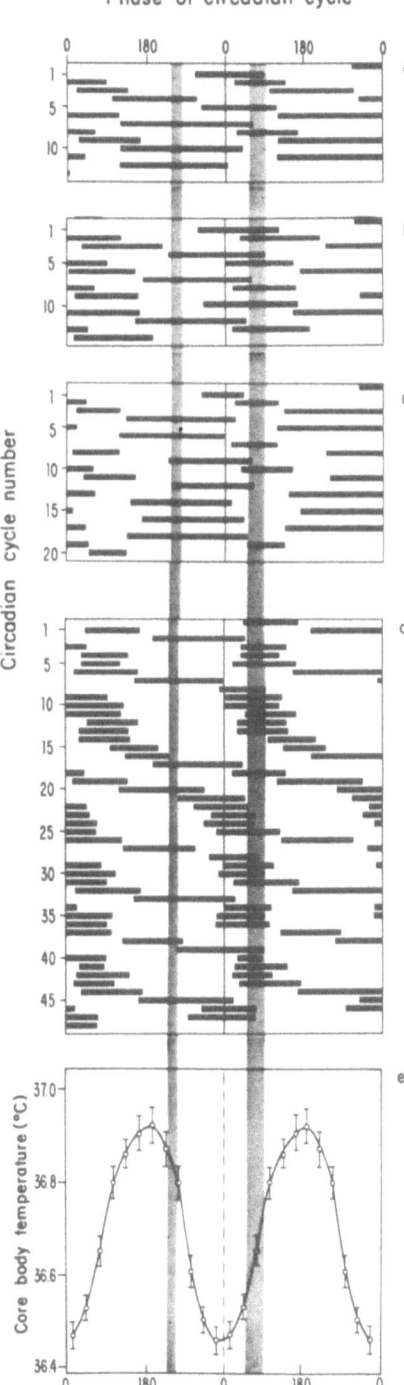

Figure 4-11. Normalized raster plots of sleep-wake records from internally desynchronized subjects. Stippled vertical bands show wake-maintenance zones in the circadian cycle. (a) Subject 3.7 (b) Subject 3.8 (c) Subject 3.9 (d) Subject 3.1.

(e) Average waveform of body temperature for the desynchronized subjects of (a-d). Wake-maintenance zones occur on steep sections of the temperature curve.

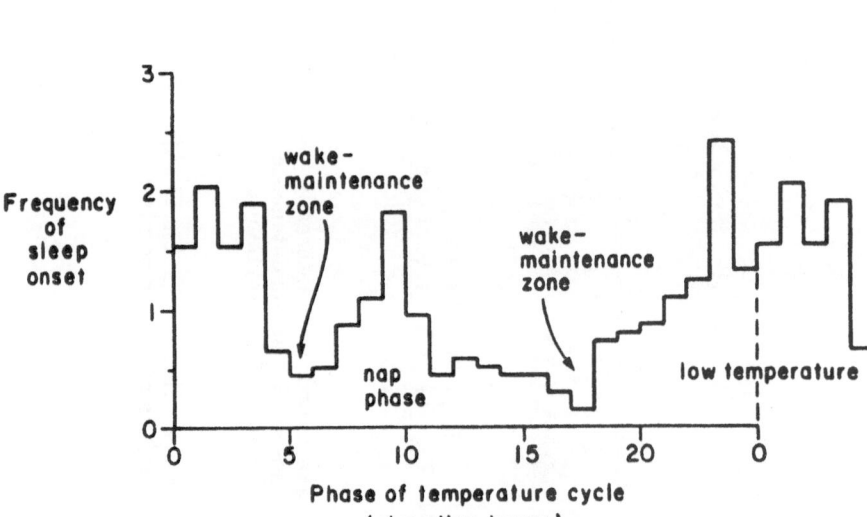

Figure 4-12. Distribution of sleep onsets selected at different phases in the circadian cycle. A frequency of 1 represents the average frequency across all phases. Approximate times of day are shown above the distribution, based on a conversion $(\phi=0) \sim$ 6-7 AM for male college students with an average habitual wake-time around 8:30 AM (Czeisler, 1985; Czeisler *et al.*, 1986).

transition is somehow actively inhibited, not just passively avoided. Several lines of evidence indicate that is indeed hard to fall asleep in the evening wake-maintenance zone (the status of the morning zone turns out to be more complicated).

4.5.2 90-Minute Day and Other Ultradian Sleep Studies

In ultradian sleep studies, researchers have examined subjects' ability to fall asleep at many times of day and night. (Carskadon and Dement, 1975, 1977, 1980; Webb and Agnew, 1975; Weitzman *et al.*, 1974; Moses *et al*, 1975; Lavie and Zomer, 1984; Lavie and Scherson, 1981).

For example, in the 90-minute day studies, subjects lived on a cycle of 30 minutes bedrest, 60 minutes enforced wakefulness, then back to bed for 30 minutes, and so on, 16 times a day, all day and night for over 5 calendar days. Figure 4-13 shows the total sleep time obtained by one subject (MA) in each of his 30 minute bedrest opportunities as well as his oral temperature upon arising. A three-point running average drawn through the raw data shows evident circadian variation. Notice that in every cycle there are certain times when the total sleep time was zero. It is amazing that the subject could not manage to fall asleep, in spite of the considerable sleep deprivation (Carskadon and Dement, 1977) induced by the grueling schedule.

A time-series analysis (Figure 4-14) reveals that both the sleep and temperature data have a period of 25.25h; thus the subject was free-running as a result of the disruptive schedule, even though no effort was made to shield subjects from time cues (Carskadon and Dement, 1975, 1980).

Total sleep time varies as a function of phase in the circadian temperature cycle. The curve in Figure 4-15 shows the median sleep time for 5 subjects, and the error bars show the middle one-third of the data in each bin (equivalent to standard error of the mean, for $N = 5$). Very little sleep is obtained between $\phi = 16$—20. This is the evening wake-maintenance zone discussed earlier, centered about 7-8h before low temperature. To reiterate an earlier point with a bit of hyperbole: whereas the free-run data showed only that subjects *do not want* to go to sleep in the evening zone, the 90-minute day data show that they *cannot*. Both "sleep preference" and "sleep ability" (Lavie and Scherson, 1981) are low during the evening zone.

On the other hand, the morning zone is absent from Figure 4-14, in contrast to the free-run results. I do not understand this reason for this discrepancy.

Other ultradian studies have detected the evening zone. Weitzman *et al.* (1974) had subjects live for 10 days on a schedule of 1h rest, 2h awake. Czeisler's (1978; 1980b, Figure 7) reanalysis of these data established that the most sleep was obtained at the temperature trough, and the least was obtained about 9h before the trough, in agreement with the 90-minute day and free-run data. Webb and Agnew (1975) studied subjects on various sleep-wake regimens, including a 3h rest, 6h enforced activity cycle which continued for 6 calendar days. The 9h cycle resulted in sleep onset times at 8 different hours of the day. The average sleep latencies showed a dramatic variation with time of day, rising from less than 5 minutes at 7 AM to a peak of 55 minutes at 10 PM. (Temperature data were not reported, but the clock times of the extrema agree with those estimated in Figure 4-12.) Webb and Agnew

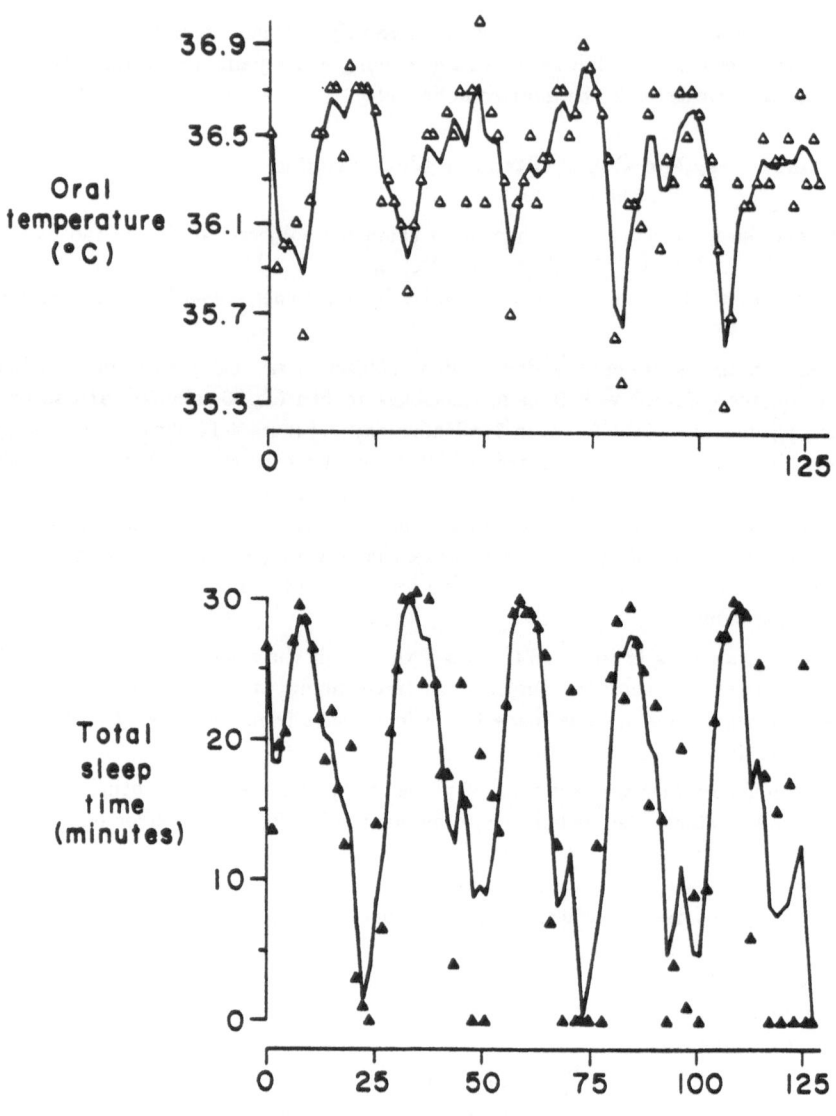

Figure 4-13. Time-series of oral temperature and time spent asleep per 30-minute bedrest for subject MA on the 90-minute day ($N = 86$ bedrest episodes and oral temperature readings). Three-point running averages (weights $1/4$, $1/2$, $1/4$) of the data are indicated by solid lines.

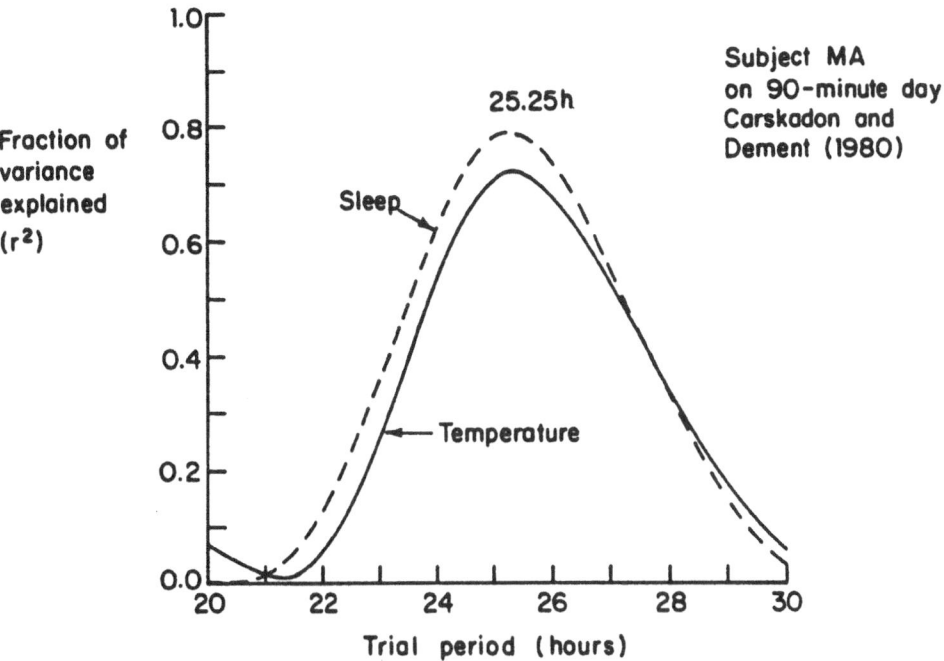

Figure 4-14. Period estimates for time series of sleep time data and oral temperature data, subject MA on the 90-minute day. (See Figure 4-13.) Temperature and sleep data were first smoothed with a five point running average. Then at a series of trial periods, a sinusoid was fit to the smoothed data by the method of least squares. The statistic r^2 was computed, representing the fraction of variance explained by the single harmonic fit. Using more harmonics or other spectral methods did not significantly alter the period estimate, which was 25.25h for both time series.

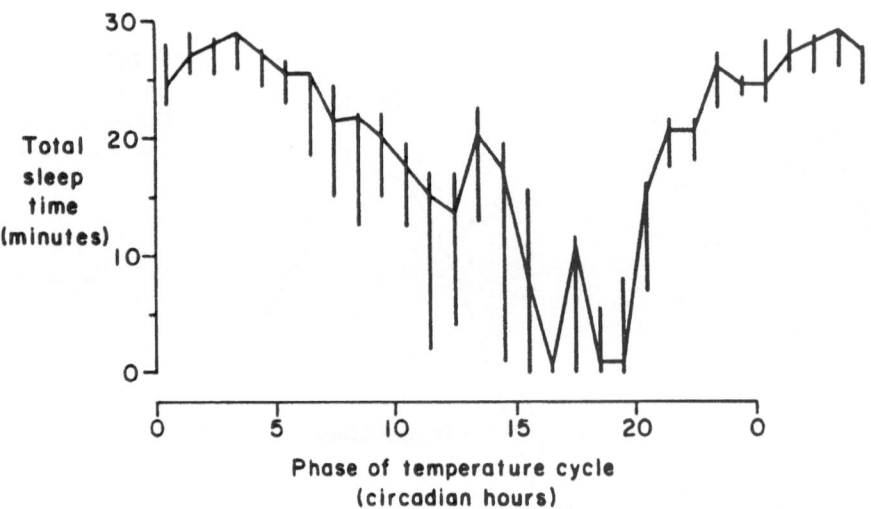

Figure 4-15. Variation of sleep time obtained per 30-minute bedrest opportunity, as a function of circadian phase at the end of the bedrest. The curve is the median for 5 subjects, and the error bars represent the central third of the data in each bin (equivalent to standard error of the mean for 5 subjects). The five subjects (Carskadon and Dement, 1980) were MA, GS, GR, WW, and MD.

The other five subjects in the study of Carskadon and Dement (1980) were omitted from the analysis because of difficulties in estimating the period or phase of the temperature time-series. (The oral temperature measurements tended to be noisy.)

(1975) describe their results as "surprising" in view of the rise in sleep latency "to a high point at the normal sleep onset time."

We are least sleepy just before our regular bedtime! The result may be paradoxical but it is consistent — in all three ultradian studies considered here, as well as in the histogram of sleep onsets in free-run, we have seen that there is a prominent minimum in sleep tendency about 7-9h before the temperature nadir. This minimum is the signature of the evening wake-maintenance zone.

4.5.3 Unintended Microsleeps During Constant Routine

Mary Carskadon has recently studied subjects on a 40h constant routine (Carskadon, 1985). During this sleep deprivation protocol, as pioneered by Mills *et al.* (1978) and systematically refined by Czeisler *et al.* (1986), subjects are kept awake for 40h in a constant supine posture. They are fed hourly aliquots of some disgusting nutrient drink, and are subjected to constant indoor light.

Czeisler's constant routine protocol has resolved a number of long-standing and fundamental questions. Because the routine eliminates the "masking" of sleep, activity, postural changes and feeding, it exposes the waveshape of endogenous rhythms. Czeisler *et al.* (1985, 1986) have used the method to pinpoint the trough of the circadian temperature rhythm, an accomplishment of enormous technical and clinical importance. Carskadon (1985) has interspersed her "multiple sleep latency tests" in constant routines, and has thereby demonstrated — finally — that the mid-day dip reflects an intrinsically biphasic sleep tendency in man and is not just a trivial consequence of having eaten a big lunch.

But Carskadon found something else, something unexpected and very intriguing. Although subjects on the constant routine are supposed to stay awake the whole time, they don't — they occasionally drop off into a "microsleep." For a few seconds the brain falls asleep and the EEG pattern changes suddenly. What Carskadon has found is that these unintended sleep episodes are most likely to occur at certain times of day (Figure 4-16). The histogram of microsleeps has local maxima at the temperature trough and nap phase, and local minima at the two wake-maintenance zones. Thus the bimodal rhythm of nodding off during sleep deprivation matches the bimodal rhythm of bedtime selection during free-run (presumably both reflect the circadian component of sleep tendency).

4.5.4 Free-Running in Society

Wollman and Lavie (1986; Lavie *et al.*, 1985) have reported a case of a man who is not blind yet is unable to entrain to the 24h world. While there have been previous reports of people free-running in society (Elliott *et al.*, 1971; Kokkoris *et al.*, 1978; Miles *et al.*, 1977; Weber *et al.*, 1980), Wollman and Lavie's patient is particularly exciting because his sleep-wake diary of four and half years contains a "hidden regularity" (Wollman and Lavie, 1986): his sleep onsets are not distributed uniformly around the clock but instead show gates and wake-maintenance zones at the times expected for healthy young people (Figure 4-17). Note the sharp minimum at 11 PM, signalling the standard location of the evening zone, with a secondary minimum near noon (the morning zone).

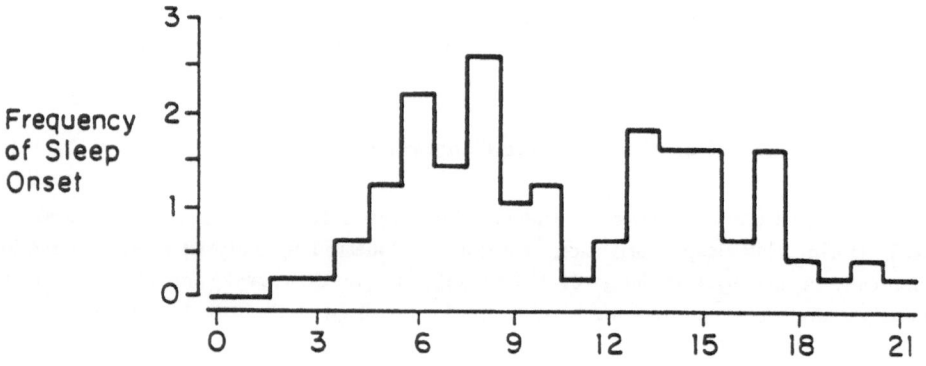

Hourly distribution of
unintended microsleeps during
constant routine
(from Carskadon 1985)

Frequency
of Sleep
Onset

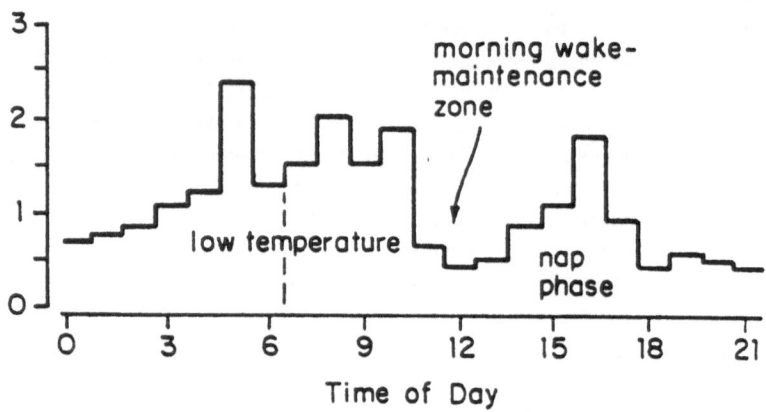

Bedtimes selected
during internal
desynchronization

morning wake-
maintenance
zone

low temperature

nap
phase

Time of Day

Figure 4-16.

(**top**): Bimodal distribution of unintended sleep episodes during the last 22h of a 40h constant routine. Frequency of 1 equals the average frequency across all bins. N = 287 sleep episodes, 16 subjects. Data from Carskadon (1985), kindly provided by Dr. Carskadon.

(**bottom**): Bimodal distribution of sleep onsets selected during desynchrony (Figure 4-12) is redrawn for comparison to microsleep data above. Circadian phases have been converted to approximate times of day by assigning 6:30 AM to low temperature (Czeisler *et al.*, 1986). The similar waveforms suggest that physiologic sleep tendency in man is bimodal.

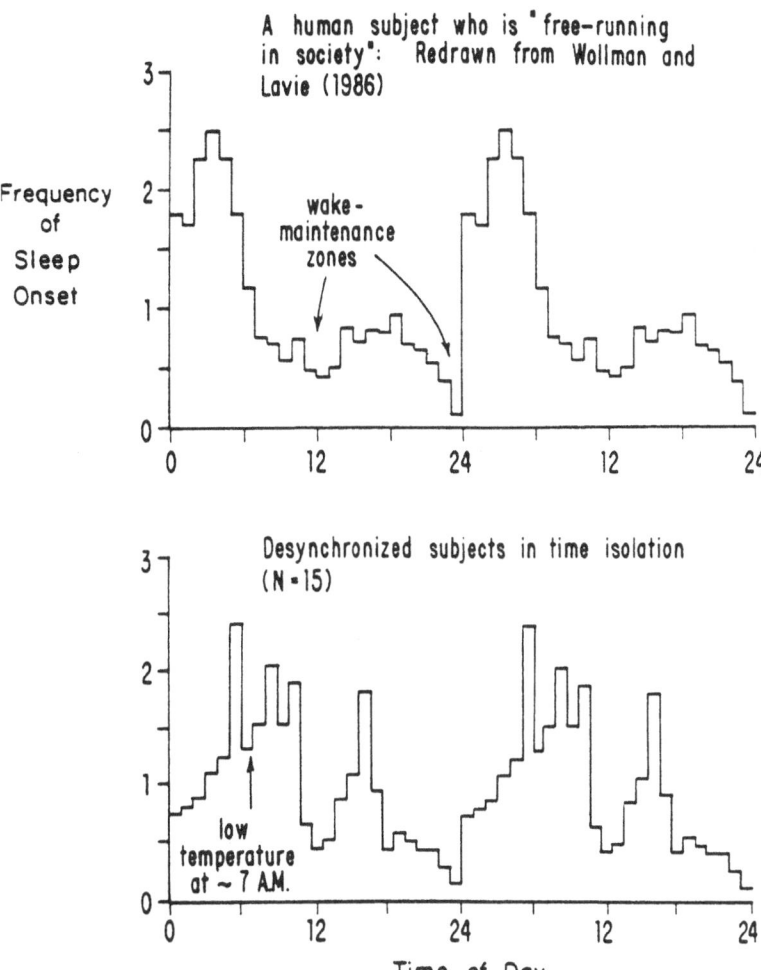

Figure 4-17. (top): Double-plotted distribution of bedtimes chosen by a patient who is unable to synchronize his sleep schedule to the 24h world, i.e. his sleep times drift around the clock. (A frequency of 1 corresponds to the mean frequency across all times of day.) His sleep onset distribution resembles that extrapolated from normal subjects who have internally desynchronized during free-run (**bottom**), suggesting that his circadian pacemaker was normally entrained to the 24h world.

Data kindly provided by M. Wollman and P. Lavie; top panel redrawn from Wollman and Lavie (1986).

The invariance and positioning of the zones suggests that the patient's temperature rhythm was successfully and normally entrained to the 24h day, even though sleep was drifting around the clock. Similarly, Wever (1979, Fig. 81, p. 148) has reported a laboratory experiment in which a subject's temperature rhythm was entrained to 24h even though his sleep-wake cycle had desynchronized. Kronauer (1984) has successfully simulated this phenomenon, a surprising result considering that his model does not assume any direct influence of zeitgebers on the temperature pacemaker. Finally, note that Wollman and Lavie's patient appears to have a different disorder from that reported by Kokkoris *et al.* (1978) — the temperature rhythm of the Kokkoris patient appears to have *desynchronized* from the 24h day, perhaps because of an excessively long intrinsic period.

4.5.5 Insomnia on a 23.5h Day

It might be argued that the evidence presented for wake-maintenance zones comes solely from experiments involving abnormal schedules, sleep deprivation or free-run. What about ordinary 24h entrainment? Do the zones operate in normal individuals under normal conditions? That question awaits careful experimental study. The prediction is that sleep onset insomnia is likely to occur when a zone impinges upon bedtime hours.

Such a case of insomnia was inadvertently induced in a healthy young subject by Fookson *et al.* (1984). In an experiment designed to probe the limits of zeitgeber entrainment, they placed a 21-year old male (PB04) on a 23.5h schedule — only a half-hour shorter than normal and unknown to the subject. During his scheduled 7.75h bedrest each day, the subject either fell asleep immediately or else he was unable to fall asleep for about 3h (Figure 4-18). He suffered from insomnia night after night, despite his increasing sleep debt. The subject complained bitterly about the imposed schedule and threatened to quit the experiment. All this from a mere half-hour shortening of his daily schedule!

The likely explanation is that the short schedule forcibly altered the subject's internal phase relations, anchoring the evening wake-maintenance zone at his scheduled bedtime. The temperature data provide an estimate of the location of the line $\phi = 0$ (Figure 4-18). The sleep data reveal the predicted zone, about 7-8h before $\phi = 0$, in which sleep onset never occurs. Note the cluster of onsets to either side of the zone; the subject either managed to fall asleep just ahead of the zone, or else had to endure its full extent before falling asleep.

The conclusion of the experiment supported the interpretation offered above. When the schedule was eventually shortened to 23.0h, the subject's temperature rhythm lost entrainment to the schedule, the zone was no longer locked to his bedtime, his insomnia disappeared and his mood brightened.

4.5.6 Clinical Implications

There may be people in the outside world who experience the same sort of insomnia as PB04, and for the same reason. This subject had an intrinsic circadian period $\tau = 24.7h$ and he had troublesome internal phase relations on a 23.5h day; by the same token, people with intrinsic periods near 25.2h living in a 24h world could well find themselves trying to fall asleep in a forbidden zone.

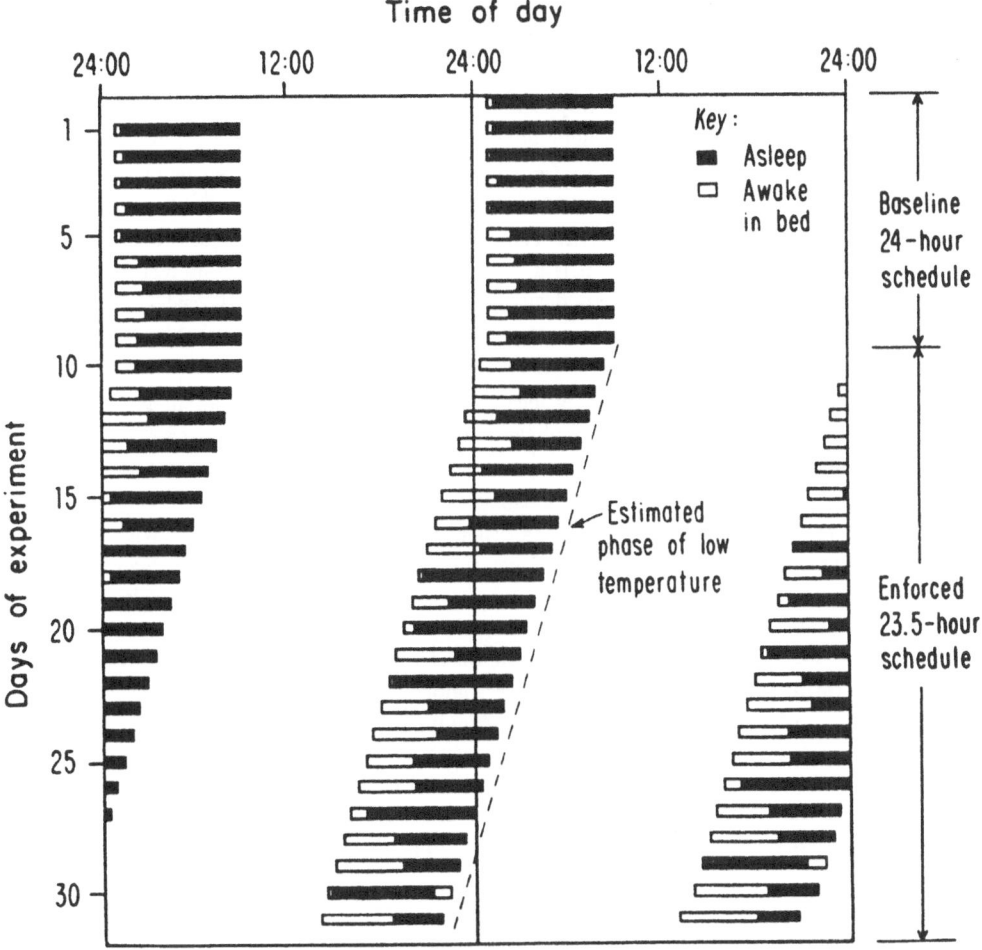

Figure 4-18. Sleep-wake raster plot of a subject (PB04) entrained to a 23.5h schedule. Sleep (black bars) was polygraphically verified. The reference phase $\phi = 0$ locates temperature minima. A zone of "forbidden" sleep onset appears in the record, coincident with the evening wake-maintenance zone observed in various other experiments (see text).

The evening wake-maintenance zone may underlie the "delayed-sleep-phase syndrome" (Czeisler *et al.*, 1981) estimated to afflict hundreds of thousands of people. People with this syndrome are able to sleep well but only if they sleep at the "wrong" time of day (e.g. 4 AM to noon). This makes it practically impossible for them to hold any job which requires alertness in the morning. Some researchers have regarded this disorder as psychopathological, and have recommended psychotherapy or behavioral conditioning as treatment. Most physicians respond to the complaint of delayed sleep-phase insomnia by prescribing sleeping pills.

Using circadian principles, Czeisler *et al.* (1981) developed a successful drug-free treatment called "chronotherapy." It consists of sequentially *delaying* the subject's sleep-wake schedule around the clock until the desired orientation is reached (Czeisler *et al*, 1981). Attempts to phase *advance* the sleep episodes were unsuccessful, probably because they required the subject to try to sleep during the evening zone.

The experiment which desperately needs to be done is a circadian phase assessment (Czeisler *et al.*, 1985) of delayed-sleep-phase patients, both before and after chronotherapy. Such an experiment would test the hypothesis that delayed-sleep-phase insomnia is due to a pernicious phasing of the evening wake-maintenance zone.

The existence of the evening zone has other interesting implications. With the zone so close to habitual bedtime, we may sometimes find ourselves trying to fall asleep when it is most difficult. The familiar insomnia on Sunday night probably results from keeping later hours on the weekend; this behavior inadvertently allows the circadian cycle and its evening zone to drift to later hours, thereby impinging on the regular weekday bedtime. For millions of people, rotating shift work schedules cause a more chronic misalignment of circadian timing, sometimes leading to insomnia when the evening wake-maintenance zone interferes with the desired bedtime. Jet lag results in temporary conflicts of this sort, particularly after eastward travel, until adaptation realigns the internal clock with the outside world, and bedtime no longer falls in the evening zone. Thus the wake-maintenance zone concept unifies these seemingly disparate disorders of sleep-scheduling.

4.6 Estimating Circadian Parameters From Sleep Data Alone

During desynchronized free-run, the oscillator driving the circadian temperature rhythm continues to modulate the sleep-wake cycle (Sections 4.1-4.5). Because of the strong residual influence of the circadian oscillator, its parameters τ and ϕ are latent in the sleep-wake record itself. Normally τ and ϕ are derived from temperature data; this section describes two procedures for estimating these circadian parameters from sleep data alone.

One method, suggested by Richard Kronauer, relies on the phase clustering of sleep onsets (Section 4.4). When sleep onsets are "clustered," their distribution is far from uniform with respect to circadian phase (Figure 4-19). Hence, when the actual distribution deviates most from uniform, the sleep onsets are most tightly clustered. One simple measure of clustering is the variance of the observed distribution of sleep onsets. If sleep onsets were distributed uniformly, the distribution would be flat and consequently its variance would be small (zero in the limit of infinitely many sleeps). When the sleep onsets cluster at only a few phases, the variance will be large due to the peaks and valleys in the distribution (Figure 4-19). The procedure then is to search a range of trial periods and select that one which maximizes the variance.

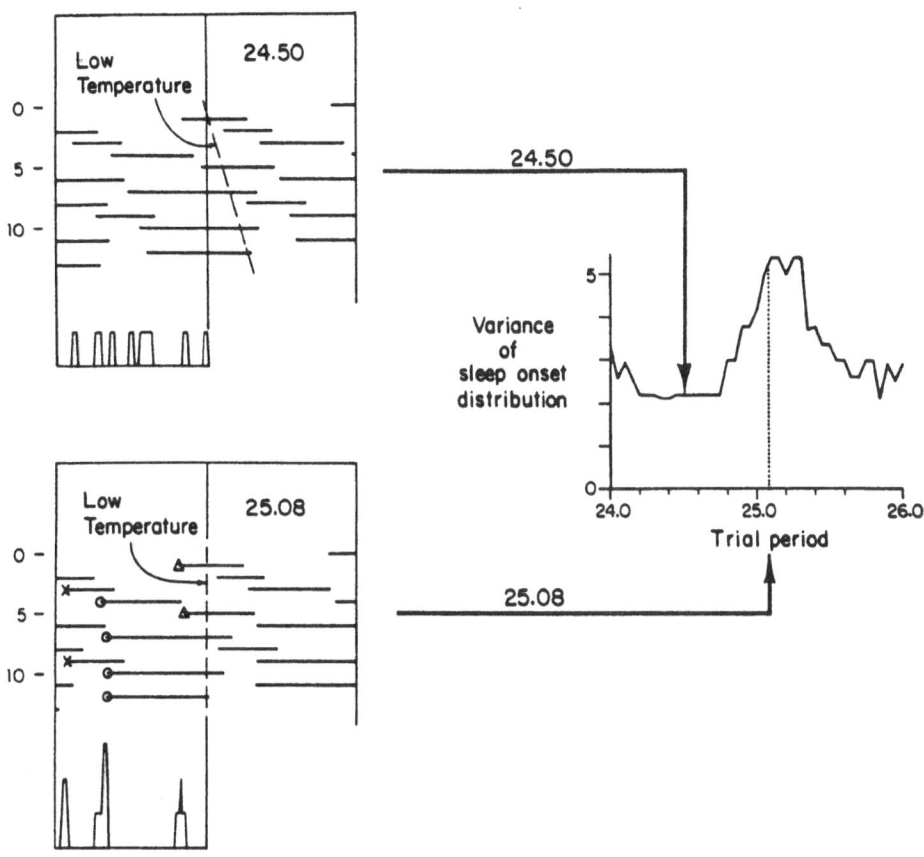

Figure 4-19. Estimate of circadian period based on maximizing the variance of the sleep onset distribution in the circadian cycle. For each trial period, a distribution is computed by counting the number of sleep onsets occurring in each of 50 bins covering the cycle. Each bin is two circadian hours wide — hence a given sleep onset will be counted in several adjacent bins. The estimated circadian period is that which maximizes sleep onset clustering, as measured by the variance of the distribution.

The method is applied to Subject 3.7 (FR03). At $\tau = 24.50$, there is poor clustering, corresponding to a low variance. At $\tau = 25.08$ (the educed temperature period), there is strong clustering into three sharp gates, yielding a variance near the maximum.

To calibrate the method I have applied it to cases of internal desynchrony where the temperature period is known directly. The estimate based on sleep onsets is found to be unbiased with a standard deviation of 0.2h (Table 4-1).

A second method (Czeisler, 1978) for estimating τ from sleep data involves the *duration* of sleep episodes, instead of their clustering. As before, one examines a range of possible τ values. For each candidate τ, sleep lengths are plotted against phase of sleep onset, where phase is computed relative to a cycle of that trial period. As Winfree (1982c, Figure 3; 1984, Figure 1) has shown, the data cloud is "a shambles" until within a narrow range of τ it abruptly aligns along the standard ramp-shaped curve (Figure 4-20). In other words, at a select period, the functional relationship is tightest; the data have minimum variance about an average curve drawn through them. (No assumption is made about what that functional relationship might be — it just happens that a ramp typically emerges.) This estimator of τ is precise to within about 0.2h. (Table 4-1)

Of course, instead of using sleep length data, similar methods could be based on prior wake length or wake-sleep cycle length (Section 4.1).

Having estimated the circadian period, one can estimate phase by searching for maximal overlap with the standard $\phi_s{:}\rho$ ramp (Section 4.1) and by locating wake-maintenance zones (Section 4.5).

As an example of these methods, consider the cave study of Jouvet *et al.* (1974) for which temperature data are unavailable. The methods indicate $\tau \sim 24.3\text{h}$ (Figure 4-21). A value of 24.27 was chosen by fine-tuning the choice of τ to produce the widest wake-maintenance zones. To determine the absolute phase, I plotted sleep length vs. arbitrary phase at $\tau = 24.27$. The data follow a ramp as expected. Aligning the sleep length data with the standard reference (Figure 4-1a) predicts a locus of $\phi = 0$ as shown in Section 3.4.

4.7 Phase-Trapping

Kronauer *et al.* (1982) introduced the term "phase-trapping" to describe a pattern in which "the sleep-wake (y) and temperature (x) rhythms have the same average period, but sleep exhibits periodic phase modulations with respect to temperature" (Kronauer and Gander, 1984). Examples which might be interpreted as phase-trapping are shown in Figure 4-22.

The last sentence is deliberately cautious because phase-trapping is controversial. Mathematically there is no issue — a weakly attracting limit cycle oscillator can certainly exhibit phase-trapping if subjected to appropriately weak periodic forcing (Stoker, 1950).

Winfree (1982b) nicely explains the controversy about phase-trapping: "The question *here* is whether humans do it [phase-trapping] on a regular basis. Several models currently entertained by workers in this area are probably incapable of phase-trapping. I would assign high priority to quantitative demonstration that this is no artifact of selective attention to noisy data, but rather a consistent regularity of many records, only heavily obscured by noise."

Possible instances of phase-trapping to be found in the data bank of Chapter 3 are subjects 3.1, 3.2, 3.4 and 3.17. Kronauer and Gander (1984) present additional examples. Some records show a few clear and regular cycles, others require more suspension of disbelief. I

Table 4-1: Estimates of Circadian Period τ

Subject	Temperature	Sleep onsets	Sleep lengths
3.1	24.55	24.40	24.55
3.2(de)	25.23	25.15	25.20
3.2(bi)	25.03	24.85	24.90
3.3	24.68	24.80	24.90
3.7	25.08	25.25	25.15
3.8	24.33	24.30	24.70
3.9	24.27	24.35	24.35

$(\tau_{\text{sleep onsets}}) - (\tau_{\text{temperature}}) = -0.01 \pm 0.14$ (mean $\pm$ S.D.)

$(\tau_{\text{sleep lengths}}) - (\tau_{\text{temperature}}) = +0.08 \pm 0.17$ (mean $\pm$ S.D.)

Table 4-1. Comparison of three methods for estimating the circadian period τ. The first estimate is based on minimum variance waveform eduction (Czeisler, 1978) of temperature, and is the "gold standard" for estimating τ. The only subjects considered here were those in which internal desynchronization occurred spontaneously, and for whom temperature eductions were available. Results for methods based on sleep onset clustering (Figure 4-19) and sleep length residuals (Figure 4-20) are listed in the third and fourth column, respectively.

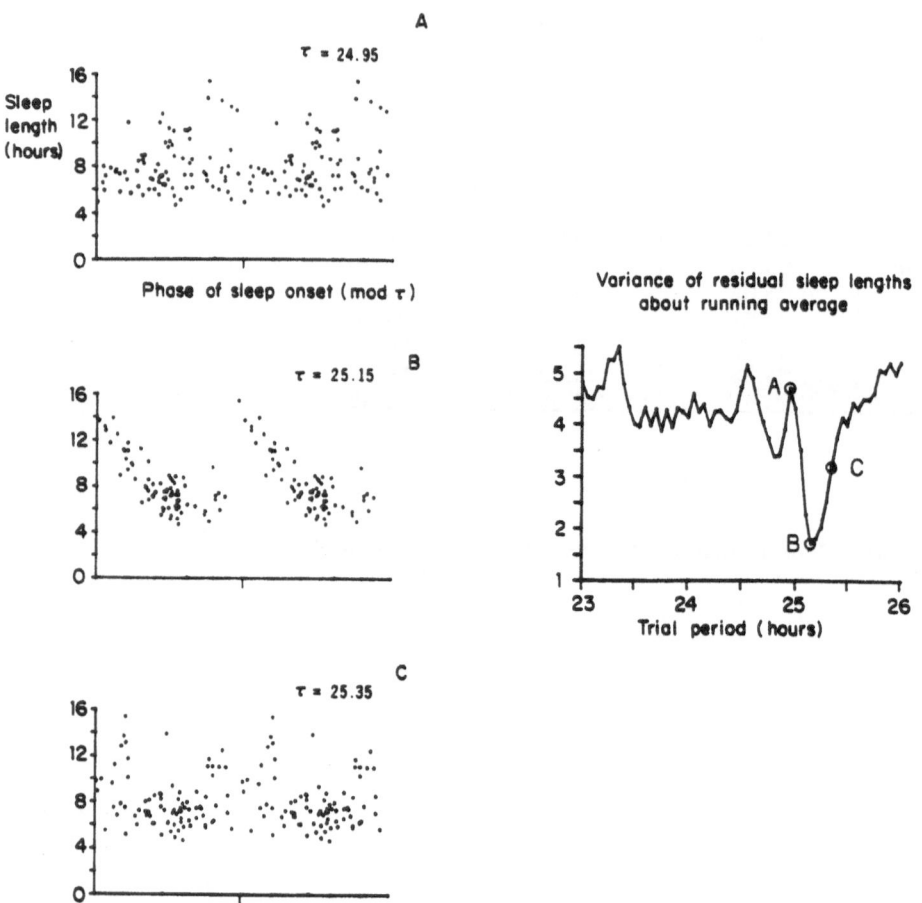

Figure 4-20. Estimate of circadian period based on minimizing the scatter of the ϕ_s:ρ relation (Czeisler, 1978; Winfree, 1982c). A running average (not shown) of the raw ϕ_s:ρ data is computed using a "raised cosine" filter of 1h full width. Residual deviations of ρ from the curve are computed for each datum, and then squared and summed over all points. This quantity is proportional to the variance of the residual sleep lengths. The estimated period is that which minimizes the variance.

The method is applied to Subject 3.2 (LD03). Data are drawn from the last 83 sleep episodes of the record (its desynchronized section). At trial periods (A) $\tau = 24.95$h or (C) $\tau = 25.35$h, the double plotted ϕ_s:ρ data cloud has no apparent structure, corresponding to a large variance. At trial period (B) $\tau = 25.15$h, the cloud forms the familiar ramp (Figure 4-1a), and its tight functional relationship yields the minimum variance of the residual sleep lengths.

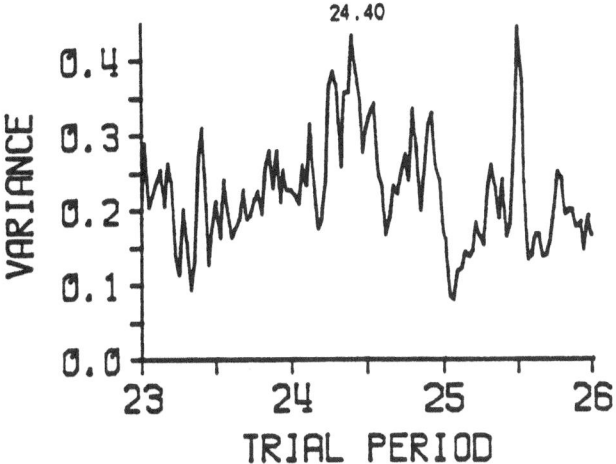

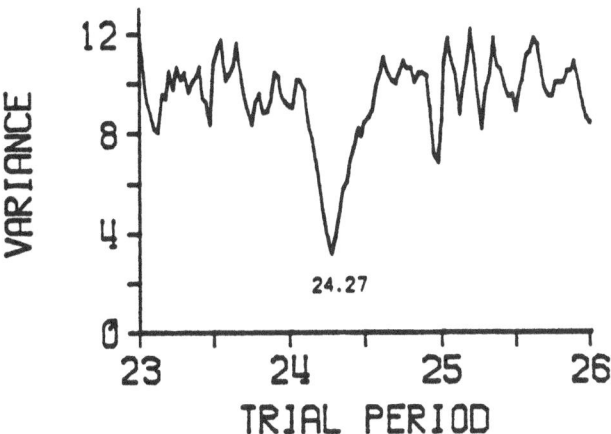

Figure 4-21. Estimates of circadian period for Subject 3.4 (Jouvet JC), for whom temperature data are unavailable. Based on sleep data alone, the methods suggest $\tau \sim 24.3$.

(top): The maximum variance of the sleep onset distribution (Figure 4-19) occurs at 24.40h.

(bottom): The minimum variance of sleep length residuals (Figure 4-20) occurs at 24.27h.

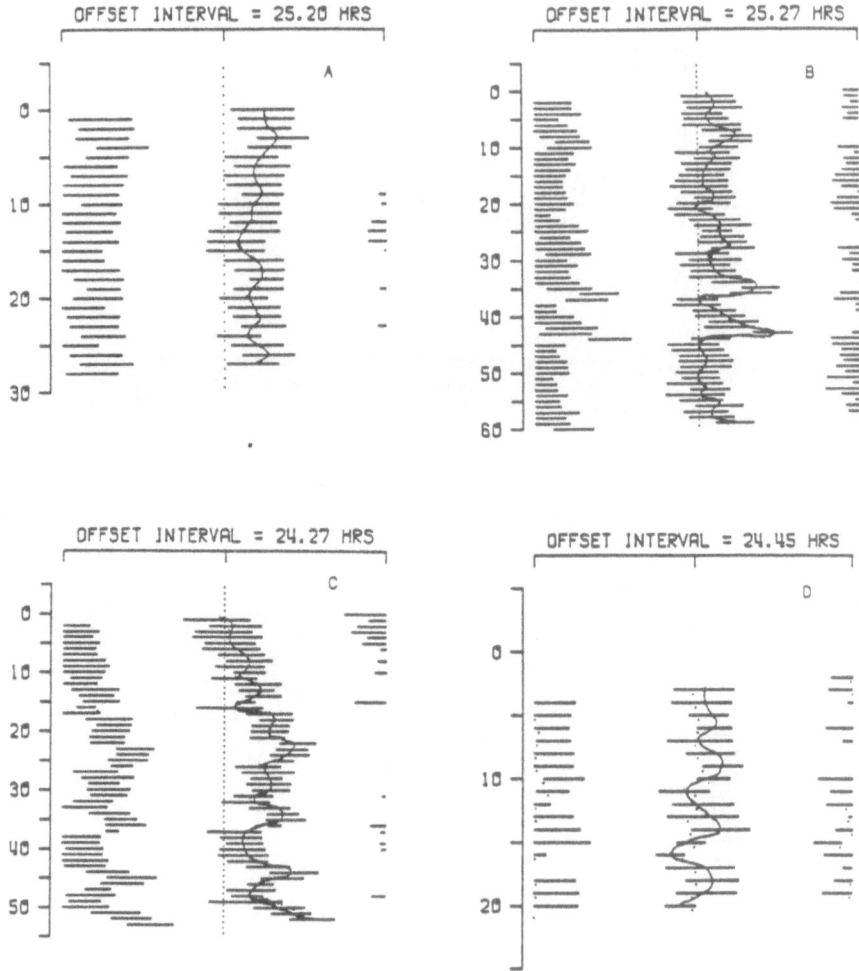

Figure 4-22. Phase-trapping in records of free-run: sleep and temperature have same average period, but an oscillatory phase relation. Offset interval is the period of the temperature cycle. In (A), (B), and (D), the raster midline locates low temperature.

(A) = Subject 3.1 (PR01); first 28 sleep episodes

(B) = Subject 3.2 (LD03); first 59 sleep episodes

(C) = Subject 3.4 (Jouvet JC); first 52 bedrests; no temperature data available

(D) = Figure 28 of Wever (1979); first 18 bedrest episodes

    Dots = temperature minima

have not given a "quantitative demonstration" in Winfree's sense, and indeed I doubt that any could be given. By its nature, phase-trapping typically occurs over a small part of parameter space. It is a delicate phenomenon poised between synchrony and desynchrony. As such it is unlikely to last long enough to allow statistical tests of periodicity.

On the other hand, an ensemble assessment may be a possible solution. As more free-run studies accumulate, enough examples may be found to establish the case for phase-trapping.

A different approach is to use computer simulations to see if noise alone can produce patterns suggestive of phase-trapping. If so then phase-trapping may have been a mirage all along.

To sum up, phase-trapping — whether real or not — is not robust enough to act as a solid test of models.

4.8 Slow Changes in Sleep-Wake Cycle Length

Czeisler (1978) noticed a fascinating similarity among several published records of sleep-wake timing during free-run. In a suggestive figure, he arranged different records along a continuum. Each stage in the orderly progression is exhibited by the four and a half month record reported by Jouvet *et al.* (1974) (Figure 4-23, reproduced from Czeisler (1978), Figure 23). In the Jouvet record the sleep-wake pattern slowly unfolds and evolves. The changing appearance of the record is tied to a gradual lengthening of the average sleep-wake cycle period. This parameter drifts from about 25h at the beginning of free-run to about 44h at the end.

These observations led Kronauer *et al.* (1982) to advance a provocative hypothesis: the intrinsic period τ_y of the hypothesized activity pacemaker lengthens during prolonged temporal isolation. According to this view, different subjects may begin at different points along the continuum of intrinsic periods — that would explain why some desynchronize immediately after release from 24h entrainment, whereas others remain internally synchronized for a month or more. Furthermore some subjects are said to show "internal phase drift" and "phase-trapping" (Section 4.7) before outright desynchronization — both phenomena are consistent with a secular lengthening of τ_y (Kronauer *et al.*, 1982; Moore-Ede *et al.*, 1982).

The long records available show that subjects do not always become more and more desynchronized, as would be expected if τ_y were to increase monotonically (Figure 4-24; compare Figure 3-1). LD04 never desynchronized in six months; Siffre desynchronized after about a month, then spontaneously regained synchrony for over two months and then lost it again; Mills DL apparently resynchronized after an initial desynchrony; so did J.P. Mairetet, one of Siffre's cave subjects (Siffre, 1972, Figure 38). As Richard Kronauer has pointed out, LD03 has an increasing activity cycle length but modulated by ~ 20 day oscillations (Figure 4-25).

As of this writing, the long-term behavior of the free-running sleep-wake cycle is mysterious. No consistent patterns have been found.

MULTI - STUDY COMPARISON OF ACTIVITY/REST CYCLE PATTERN PLOTS

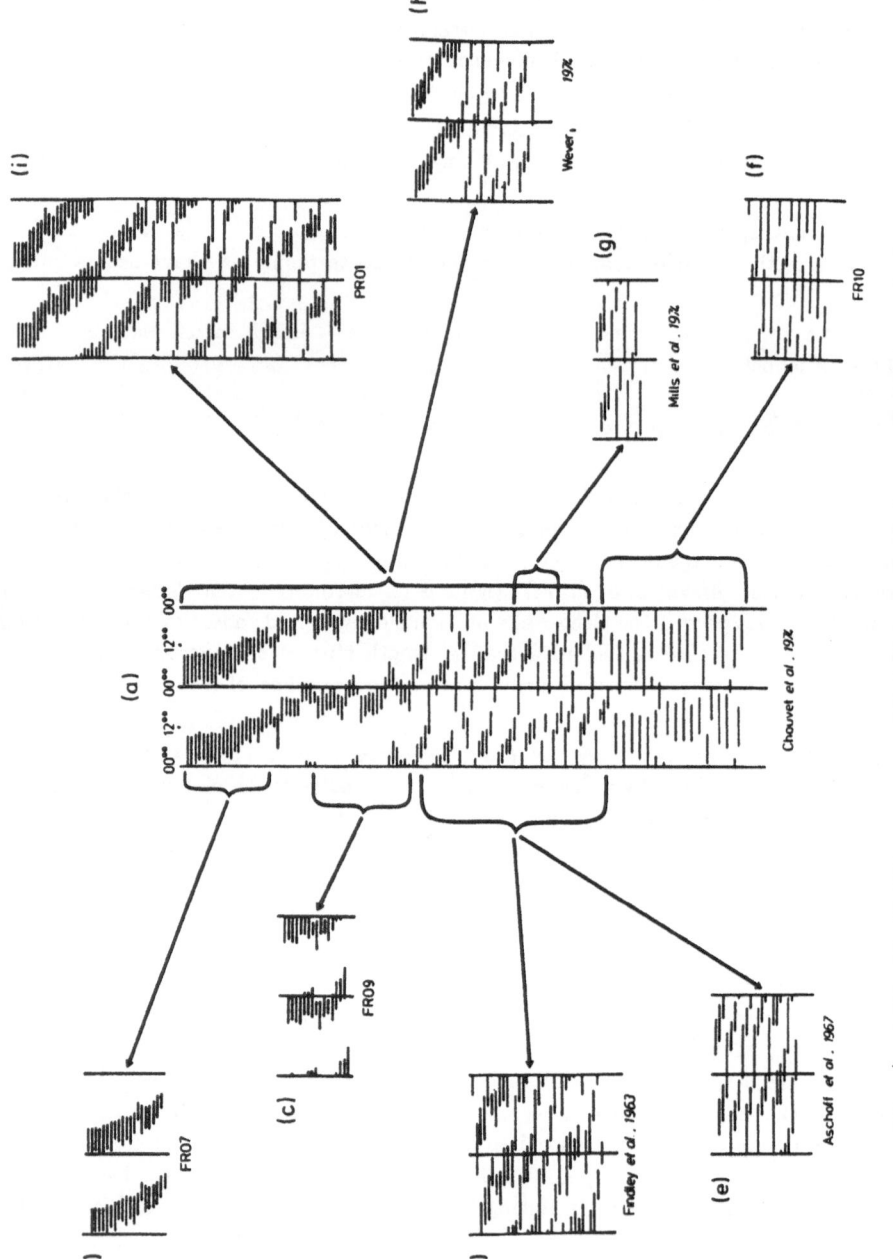

Figure 4-23. Similarities among published records of sleep-wake patterns during free-run. (Reproduced from Czeisler (1978), Figure 23, with permission.)

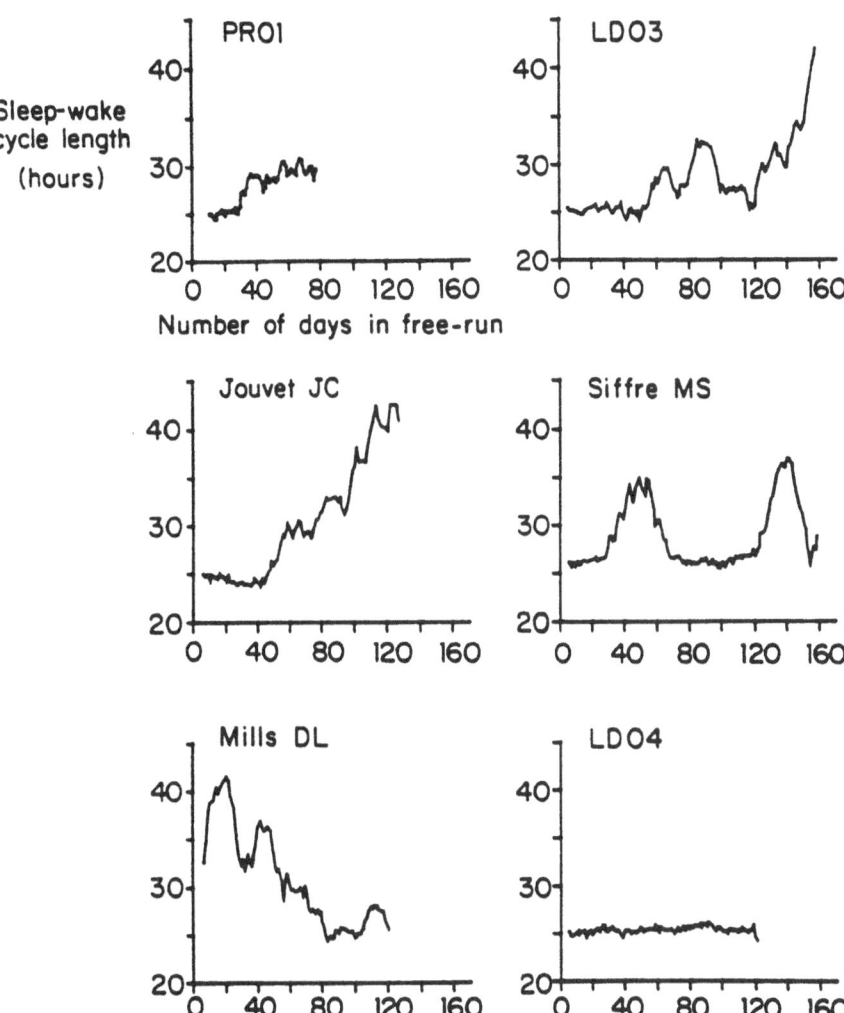

Figure 4-24. Long-term behavior of the sleep-wake cycle length during free-run. For each sleep-wake cycle, an "individual cycle length" is defined as the time interval between successive sleep onsets. To elucidate secular variations of cycle length, an 11-point running average (equal weights) of individual cycle lengths is shown here. No average was computed for the five cycles at either end of the record.

PR01 = Subject 3.1; Jouvet JC = Subject 3.4; Mills DL = Subject 3.16; LD03 = Subject 3.2; Siffre MS = Subject 3.5; LD04 = Subject 3.17.

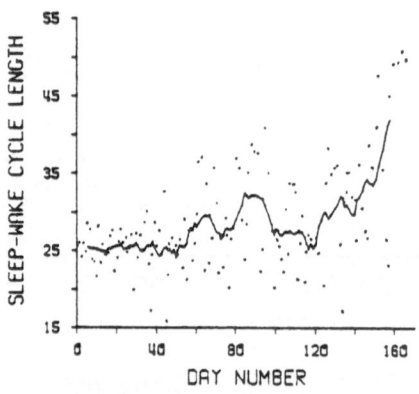

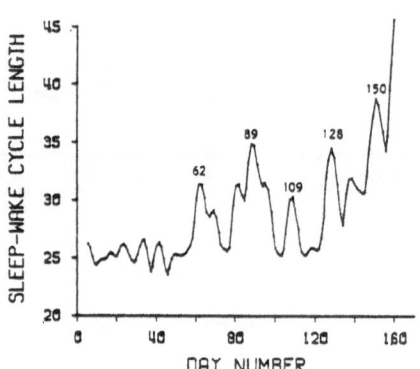

Figure 4-25. Long-term variations of sleep-wake cycle length of LD03 (Subject 3.2). Day 0 is the first day of free-run (*not* the first day of the experiment, as in Figures 2-1, 2-2; see instead the raster plot of free-run in Section 3.2).

(top): Dots are raw data of individual cycle lengths, defined as time interval between consecutive sleep onsets. The curve is an 11-point running average, with all points in the average weighted equally, as in Figure 4-24.

(bottom): Another 11-point running average, except now with a bell-shaped smoothing kernel instead of the "boxcar" above. The relative weights in the kernel are binomial, i.e.,

$$ w_n = \frac{1}{2^{10}} \frac{10!}{(10-n)!\,n!} \quad , \qquad n = 0,1,2,\cdots,10 $$

Numbers indicate days on which cycle length is a local maximum. Note the 20-25 day modulation revealed by the binomial kernel.

4.9 Miscellany and Missing Patterns

Certain generalizations about sleep-wake and temperature data are comparably reliable to those mentioned earlier, but they do not fit neatly into any previous category. Such results are described briefly in this section. Also, there is an interesting class of missing patterns — these are predicted by various models but are noticeably absent from real data.

4.9.1 Compromise Period

During internal synchronization, the temperature rhythm and the sleep-wake cycle have the same average period. When desynchronization occurs, the temperature cycle typically shortens but by much less than the sleep-wake cycle lengthens. Because the synchronized period is between these two extremes, it is called the compromise period.

The point is that the temperature cycle reliably shortens after synchrony is lost — Wever (1979) has found $\Delta \tau = -0.70 \pm 0.38h$, which is significantly different from zero with $p < 0.001$. Similar results are obvious in records where there is synchrony before desynchronization occurs, e.g. Wever (1979, Figs. 27, 36).

Some authors (Kawato et al., 1982; Daan et al., 1984) have ignored this consistent shortening, claiming it is a relatively small change compared to the 5-15h lengthenings in the sleep-wake cycle. Others have seen it as offering fundamental insights: Kronauer et al. (1982) interpret the compromise period as a reflection of the *mutual* coupling of sleep-wake and temperature oscillators, whereas Eastman (1984) ascribes the period change after desynchrony to light-induced phase shifts of the temperature oscillator.

Note that the compromise period can change over the course of a record — for example, see Section 3.5. Interpreted through the model of Daan et al. (1984) (Section 5.6), this finding implies a change in circadian period τ ; whereas in the model of Kronauer et al. (1982) (Section 5.3), it could be explained as a change in $\hat{\tau}_y$, consistent with the postulated lability of this parameter.

To sum up, the shortening of the temperature period after desynchrony is real. Modellers have to confront it, sooner or later. Although the change is small and has little effect on computer simulations, its conceptual significance should not be pooh-poohed. Something — probably either light or sleep itself — influences the circadian pacemaker differently during synchrony and desynchrony.

4.9.2 Sex Differences and Correlation Structure of Synchrony

In a thorough study of 27 internally synchronized men and women, Wever (1984a) reported two interesting sex differences. Women $(N = 11)$ had significantly larger sleep fractions $(0.39 \pm 0.04$ vs. $0.33 \pm 0.04)$ and shorter synchronized periods $(24.75 \pm 0.48$ h vs. 25.22 ± 0.56 h) compared to men. For some unknown reason, women seem to need more sleep then men, at least during synchronized free-run.

The correlations between the lengths of consecutive sleep and wake episodes reflect an important asymmetry between sleep and wake. Wever (1984a) found that longer wake is followed by shorter sleep, with a correlation coefficient of $r = -0.53 \pm 0.22$. In contrast, sleep length and following wake length were not significantly correlated $(r = -0.12 \pm 0.21)$. Wake-wake and sleep-sleep correlations were also essentially zero. Thus the key correlation is that between wake and subsequent sleep, and it is negative (cf. Section 4.2).

4.9.3 The Snowstorm: Unpredictability of Wake Length

Results from desynchronized subjects echo the above-mentioned lack of correlation between sleep length and subsequent wake length. Indeed one of the greatest puzzles of desynchrony is: What sequence of prior measurements are needed to predict how long a desynchronized subject will stay awake? If instead we were to ask, what predicts the length of a sleep episode, then a *single* measurement suffices for good prediction: sleep length depends on the phase of the circadian cycle at bedtime (Section 4.1.1), except for the ~ 5h band of phases where sleep length is bimodal.

In comparison, the length of a wake episode is notoriously difficult to predict. Neither the phase of wake-up nor the prior sleep or wake length is adequate (Figure 4-26). Winfree (1984) has applied computer graphics to the data of Jouvet JC (Section 3.4) in his search for regularity in sleep onset times. Distinguishing between the situation for sleep and wake, he writes (1982c):

> · · · a plot of wake-up phase above prior sleep onset phase is quite orderly, even including a substantial gap in which wake-up seldom occurs spontaneously. But the corresponding plot of *sleep*-onset phase above prior wake-up phase more resembles a snowstorm. In contrast, contemporary models seem to require comparable regularity in both plots.

Quantifying Unpredictability

Richard Kronauer has indicated some ways to quantify the notions of "regularity" or "predictability" in onset phase vs. duration plots like Figure 4-26a or Figure 4-1a. Divide the circadian cycle into, say, 25 bins. Let λ_i and σ_i be the mean and standard deviation of the lengths of episodes beginning in bin i, where $i = 1, 2, ..., 25$. Then σ_i measures in hours the absolute predictability in bin i, and $p_i = \sigma_i / \lambda_i$ is a dimensionless measure of the fractional predictability. An overall index P of predictability is defined by taking a weighted average across all bins:

$$P = \sum_{i=1}^{25} n_i p_i \bigg/ \sum_{i=1}^{25} n_i$$

where n_i is the number of episode onsets in bin i.

A plot of average episode length λ against circadian phase of onset reveals a striking difference between sleep and wake: the average sleep durations (Figure 4-27a) depend much more strongly on onset phase than do the wake durations (Figure 4-27b), which are virtually independent of phase. Figure 4-27c shows that for sleep duration, the standard deviation σ_i is ~ 2h, except in the bimodal region $\phi_s \sim 6$–10, where $\sigma_i \sim 6$h. The weighted average

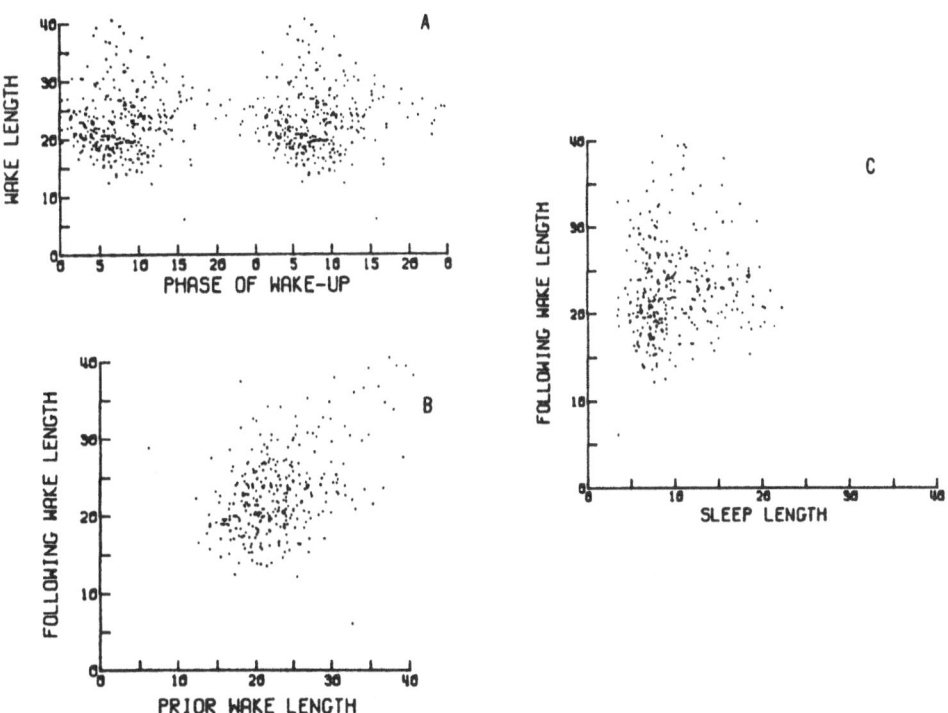

Figure 4-26. Pooled data from subjects 3.1 – 3.15, showing that the length of a wake episode is difficult to predict, given only the circadian phase of wake-up or the durations of prior sleep or waking.

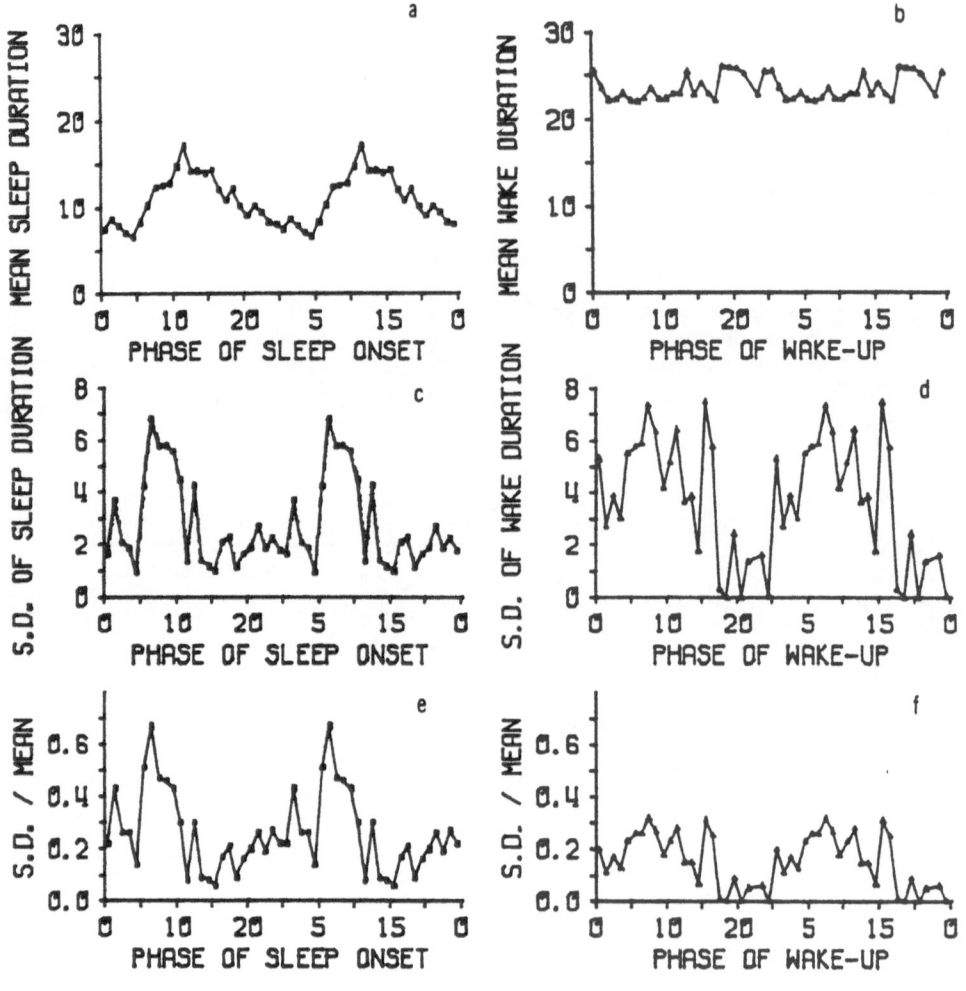

Figure 4-27. Mean duration, standard deviation (s.d.) and s.d./mean for sleep and wake episodes, as functions of circadian phase of episode onset. Compare (a), (c), (e) to Figure 4–1a, and (b), (d), (f) to Figure 4–26A.

across all phases is $\sigma = 3.3$h. In contrast, for wake (Figure 4-27d) the average $\sigma \sim 5.2$h. In terms of *absolute* duration, wake is therefore about 1.6 times less predictable than sleep. (The zero values between $\phi = 17-25$ reflect only the scarcity of awakenings in this zone (Section 4.3) and contribute little weight to the average σ.)

However, on a *percentage* basis, the roles are reversed — sleep duration is less predictable than wake duration (Figure 4-27e,f). Standard deviations for both tend to be $\sim 20\%$ of the mean, but the sleep data suffer a large percent unpredictability in the bimodal region ($p_i \sim 0.5$ for $\phi_s = 6-10$). For sleep, the weighted average of standard deviations as a fraction of the mean satisfy $P = 0.28$; for wake, $P = 0.22$.

In summary: in terms of *absolute* prediction of phase at the end of the episode, sleep is about 1.6 ($\sim 5.2/3.3$) times more predictable than wake. In terms of how the episode contributes to an ability to predict the *percent* accuracy of cycle length, wake is about 1.3 ($\sim 0.28/0.22$) times more predictable than sleep.

One final measure of predictability incorporates the disparate degrees of circadian modulation in the sleep as opposed to the wake duration data. For sleep, but *not* for wake, a knowledge of onset phase significantly improves our prediction of the episode duration, above and beyond that afforded by a knowledge of the overall mean. The relevant numerical index here is the "process r^2." It measures the fraction of the observed variance accounted for by the average "signal," and is defined as follows: let d be the vector of episode durations in Figure 4-1a or 4-26a, and let λ be the estimated signal (as in Figure 4-27a,b, where λ is a piecewise-linear function of onset phase.) Then $e = d - \lambda$ is a vector of "residuals" or deviations from the estimated signal λ. The process r^2 is defined by

$$r^2 \;=\; 1 - \frac{\mathrm{Var}(e)}{\mathrm{Var}(d)}$$

where "Var" denotes sample variance. The resultant values are

$$r^2 = 0.37 \qquad \text{(sleep)}$$
$$r^2 = 0.03 \qquad \text{(wake)}.$$

Hence, onset phase accounts for an order of magnitude more variance in the case of sleep, as opposed to wake! This is the sense intended when we say henceforth that wake duration is "relatively unpredictable".

As we shall see in Chapters 6 and 7, nearly all the available models fail to capture the asymmetry observed here between sleep and wake. The missing phase modulation in the wake data (Figure 4-27b) is a stringent test of models.

The Role of Cognition and Free Will

The problem associated with the prediction of wake length has sometimes been attributed to free will: Humans can consciously control their spontaneous bedtime (and therefore their wake duration) more than their moment of awakening (Eastman, 1984; Winfree, 1984, Moore-Ede *et al.*, 1982; Enright, 1984). Those who subscribe to this line of reasoning emphasize cognitive interactions: The subject is trying to "be good" and defers bedtime in a mistaken effort to obey the usual instructions not to nap (Mrosovsky, 1986; Zulley and Campbell, 1985); or the subject wants to postpone the rigmarole of putting on the EEG electrodes before retiring to bed; or the subject is reading a good book and wants to stay up late. According to this view, spontaneous internal desynchronization has been observed only in humans precisely because we are the only animals capable of the requisite "cognitive interactions" with the free-run protocol. So it is hardly surprising that the timing of sleep onset is unpredictable.

Against this view, Czeisler and Weitzman (in General Discussion, Moore-Ede and Czeisler, 1984) have pointed out that it is the entire structure of the day, and not just its end, which changes during internal desynchronization; "the time between waking up and having breakfast might be 6 or 8h" (Czeisler, in Moore-Ede and Czeisler, 1984, p. 209).

In the same vein, Aschoff *et al.* (1984) have recently reviewed the organization of mealtimes during both synchrony and desynchrony. They found that as soon as desynchronization occurred, the time between wake-up and lunch increased by about 4h (from 7h to 11h). They concluded that the lengthening of the cycle is accompanied by a stretching of other intervals, such as lunch to dinner or dinner to bedtime, which are related to metabolic processes. They also make the interesting remark that on long days the subjects neither eat twice as much as normal, nor do they lose as much weight as might be expected — thus suggesting a slowing of metabolism.

Finally, the argument which emphasizes cognitive interactions is defeatist. The same defeatist reasoning incorrectly suggests that the length of a sleep episode should be equally unpredictable — it depends on dream content, hunger, problems on the mind, sleep position, pajama constriction and so on. When the key to the data is found, wake durations may turn out to be as predictable as sleep duration.

But maybe the cognitive argument contains some truth — to check it, future studies should include no instructions to the subject about napping. Also, any way to simplify the attachment of EEG electrodes would help lessen the presumed cognitive interactions surrounding bedtime.

4.10 Napping and Split Sleep

All previous sections of this chapter have concentrated on free-running subjects who internally desynchronized with a *lengthening* of the sleep-wake cycle. Besides desynchrony with long τ_{SW}, and internal synchrony, two other sleep-wake patterns have been observed in free-run: "napping" with $\tau_{SW} \sim 12-14$h and "split sleep" with $\tau_{SW} \sim 18-20$h. As Richard Kronauer has pointed out, these patterns account for those that Wever (1979) describes as desynchronization with a *shortening* of the sleep-wake cycle.

Weitzman *et al.* (1982) studied the free-run behavior of two elderly subjects who habitually napped once a day. (FR11 and FR19; see Sections 3.18 and 3.19.) In free-run, their records (Figure 4-28) show one short nap, and one longer sleep episode in each circadian cycle. Note that as the nap and sleep drift across the temperature cycle, reflecting internal

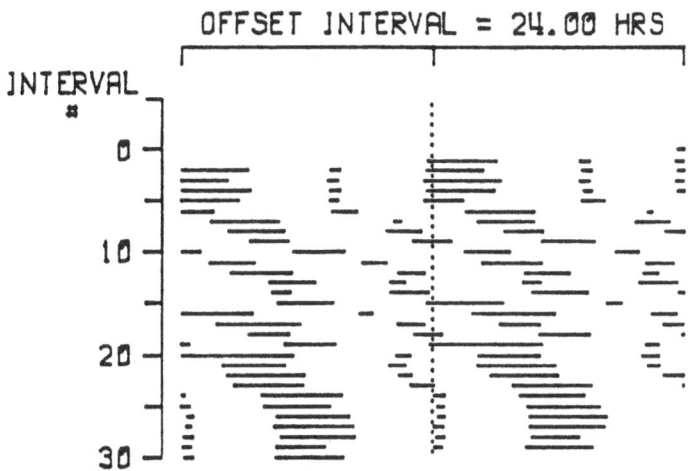

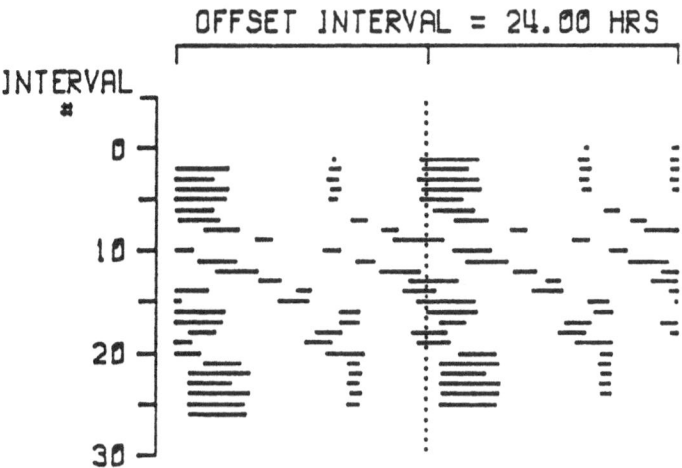

Figure 4-28. Sleep-wake raster plots of elderly nappers. **(Top):** FR11 (Section 3.18) and **(bottom):** FR19 (Section 3.19). Note both subjects were entrained to 24h before and after the free-run.

desynchronization, the naps lengthen and the sleeps shorten, until naps become sleeps and *vice versa*. This exchange reflects the circadian modulation of sleep length that occurs even in napping subjects (see below). Toward the end of the record, both subjects seemed to re-synchronize spontaneously.

In contrast to napping, a split sleep pattern (Figure 4-29) has been observed only in young subjects (Sections 3.20-22). A more precise name would be "occasional split sleep pattern," since this phenomenon is characterized by two long naps per circadian cycle, interspersed between cycles with one consolidated sleep episode. These naps are called split sleeps because on the raster plot (Figure 4-29) they bracket the middle of the ordinary consolidated sleeps and thus appear to be split versions of it.

The alternation between the split and consolidated modes of sleep follows no obvious temporal pattern. It is as if the subjects can easily switch back and forth between consolidated and split sleep. Such a phenomenon deserves further study, because it could have practical implications for the design of work schedules. Richard Kronauer has suggested that a night shift worker could take 4h naps before and after his job during the week (split sleep mode), and then follow the schedule of his family on weekends (consolidated mode). A similar schedule has been successfully adopted in a military context (see Nicholson *et al.*, 1984). The more usual alternative of one major sleep episode in the morning after work is less convenient because of daytime noise and more stressful because of the difficult shifts of the circadian system attempted during weekends.

There are two obvious differences between the nappers (Figure 4-28) and the split sleepers (Figure 4-29). One of these is happenstance while the other is important. The nappers happened to internally desynchronize while the split sleepers did not. But the *essential* distinction is that the relative durations of the nap/sleep pair are *more asymmetrical* for nappers than for split sleepers.

Sleep Length, Prior Wake Length, Cycle Length and Circadian Phase

The pooled data of subjects 3.18-3.22 are now analyzed in the manner of Sections 4.1 and 4.2. A ramp-shaped relationship (Figure 4-30) emerges once again between sleep length and the circadian phase of sleep onset. Note the key differences between Figure 4-1a and Figure 4-30: here, durations are shorter because the subjects are nappers and split sleepers, and the vertical section of data where sleep length is double-valued occurs near $\phi_s = 14-15$, not $\phi_s = 9-10$ as before.

The scatterplot of sleep length (ρ) and prior wake length (α) contains a pair of diagonally sloping clouds (Figure 4-31), in each of which the α:ρ cross-correlation is negative. Thus Figure 4-31 is qualitatively reminiscent of the earlier Figure 4-2. Note that only the split sleepers ever sample the upper cloud, where $\tau_{SW} \sim 25$h. This cloud also corresponds to the SHORT cloud of Figure 4-2, which characterizes ordinary internal synchrony.

Prior wake length (Figure 4-32) depends on the circadian phase of sleep onset, reminiscent of Figure 4-1b. Prior wake length rises monotonically and becomes double-valued near $\phi_s = 20$. When these data are added to the corresponding points of Figure 4-30, a square-wave plot of wake-sleep cycle length is obtained (Figure 4-33; cf. Figure 4-1c). The cycle

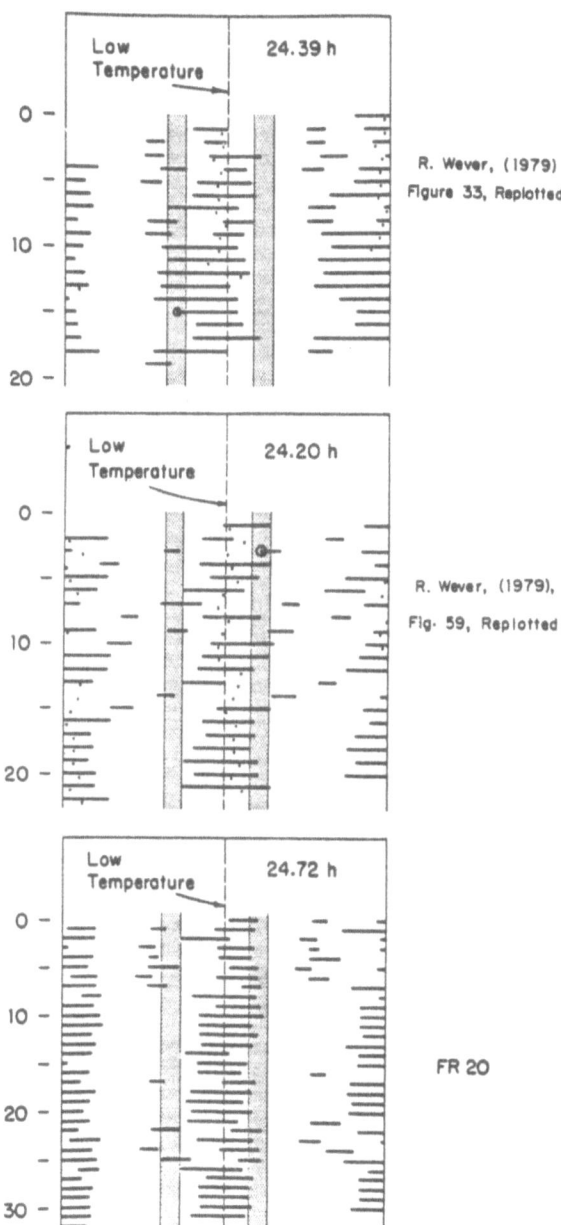

Figure 4-29. Split sleep patterns: cycles with consolidated sleeps are interspersed with cycles containing two short sleeps. The pair of short sleeps are often symmetrically poised about a line through the middle of the consolidated episodes. For more details, see Section 3.20-3.22.

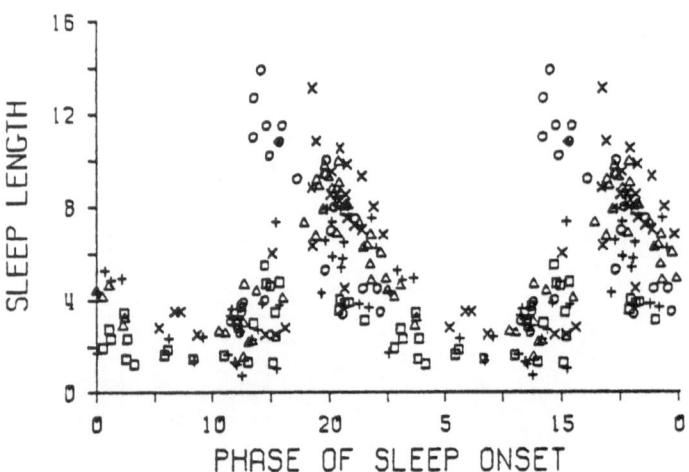

Figure 4-30. Sleep length in napping and split-sleep patterns depends on the phase of the circadian cycle at bedtime. (Pooled data from Subjects 3.18-3.22). Symbols: box = Subject 3.18; cross = 3.19; triangle = 3.20; circle = 3.21; x = 3.22.

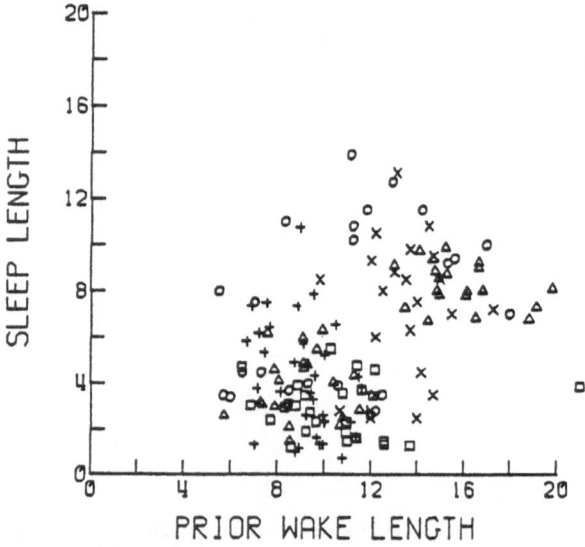

Figure 4-31. Scatterplot of sleep length and prior wake length, for Subjects 3.18-3.22. (Symbols as in Figure 4-30.)

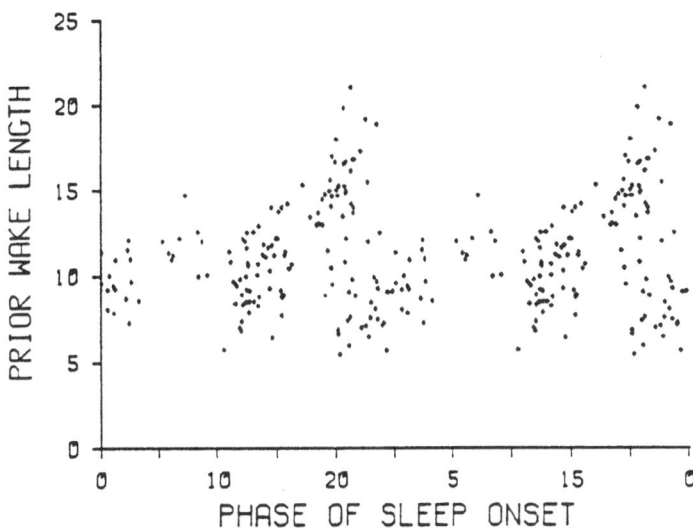

Figure 4-32. Prior wake length in napping and split-sleep patterns depends on circadian phase of sleep onset. (Pooled data, subjects 3.18-3.22.)

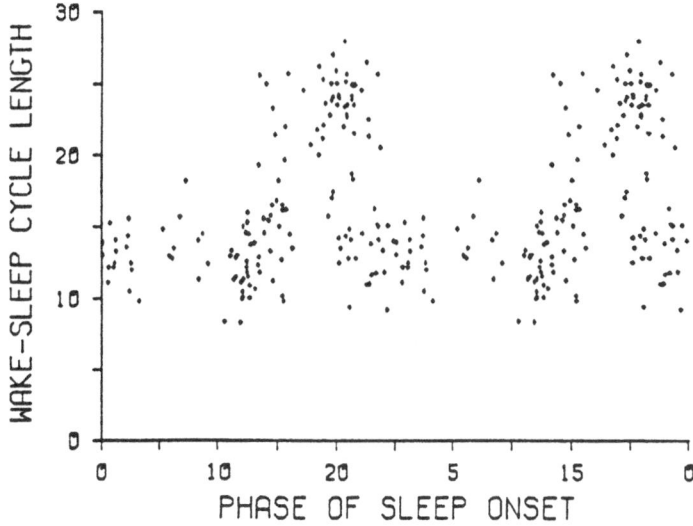

Figure 4-33. Wake-sleep cycle length in napping and split-sleep patterns depends on circadian phase of sleep onset. (Pooled data, subjects 3.18-3.22.)

lengths cluster about $\tau_{SW} \sim 24h$ and $\tau_{SW} \sim 13h$.

Timing of Sleep Onset and Wake-Up

A histogram of sleep onsets (Figure 4-34) provides another striking correspondence of napper/split sleeper data with that of desynchronized subjects. As in Figure 4-12, there is a bimodal distribution with local minima at $\phi_s \sim 5$ and $\phi_s \sim 16-18$; that is, precisely at the wake-maintenance zones documented for long τ_{SW} desynchronies (Section 4.5). (In fact it was these observations that led Kronauer to the discovery of the zones in the first place.) However, note that the major peak ($\phi_s \sim 20$) occurs earlier here than in desynchronized subjects. It is due to consolidated *synchronized* sleep episodes in the subjects of Figure 4-29. A similar bimodal distribution of sleep onsets for free-running nappers has been reported by Zulley and Campbell (1985).

In contrast to Figure 4-5, the distribution of wake-ups is bimodal (Figure 4-35), because of the presence of short naps. However, there is again a zone of forbidden waking centered at $\phi_w = 22-23$, and a strong tendency for awakening to occur on the rising limb of the temperature cycle. In fact, so many awakenings occur at $\phi_w = 4-5$ that the minimum in the distribution at $\phi_w = 8-13$ should be regarded as an artifact, due to a lack of subjects still asleep before these phases.

4.11 Summary: The Basic Patterns of Internal Desynchrony

The empirical generalizations presented here are intended as a telegraphic summary of the Chapter. The statements are based on my analysis of 355 sleep-wake cycles pooled from 15 internally desynchronized subjects; for finer details, see Table 3-1 and the individual records in Chapter 3.

Beneath each rule is a reference to the relevant section of this chapter.

1. Circadian phase of sleep onset ϕ_s predicts the length of the subsequent sleep episode. The average curve is a descending ramp, double-valued near phase $\phi_s = 8-9$. In other words, sleeps begun about 8-9 hours after the temperature trough may be either short or very long. (Section 4.1.1)

2. Circadian phase of sleep onset predicts the length of the prior wake episode. The average curve is an ascending ramp, double-valued near $\phi_s = 19-20$. (Section 4.1.2)

3. There is no significant correlation between the deviations of unrestricted sleep length and prior wake length from their circadian phase-adjusted mean curves. (Section 4.2.2)

4. Circadian phase of sleep onset predicts the wake-sleep cycle length. The average curve is a square wave. (Section 4.1.3)

5. The average co-variation of sleep length and prior wake length forms a two-branched curve. On each branch, the longer subjects stay awake, the shorter they sleep afterwards. (Section 4.2.1)

6. The distribution of wake-ups is a unimodal function of circadian phase, with almost all the awakenings during the rising part of the temperature cycle. Spontaneous wake-up in

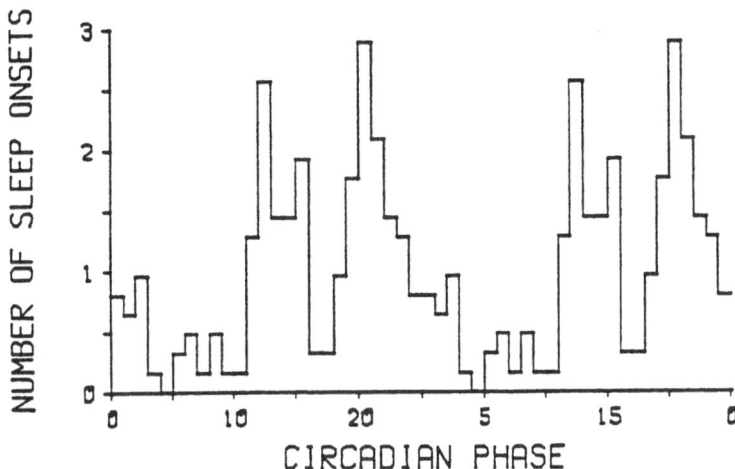

Figure 4-34. Distribution of sleep onsets in the circadian cycle, pooled data
from nappers (Subjects 3.18, 3.19) and split-sleepers (Subjects 3.20-3.22). A
frequency of 1 corresponds to the average across all phases.

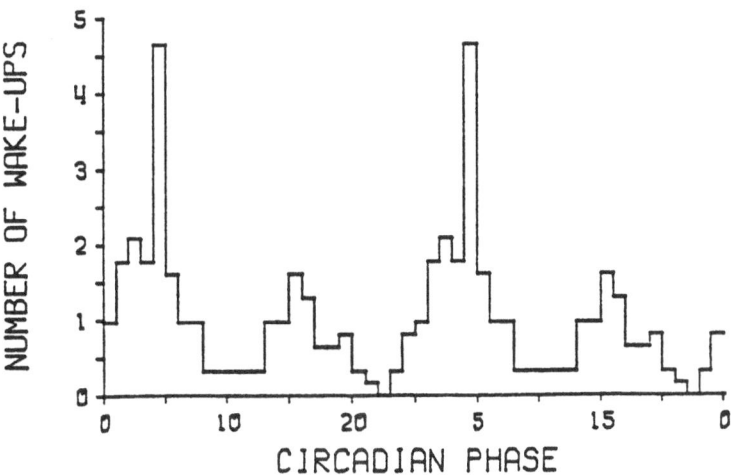

Figure 4-35. Distribution of wake-ups in the circadian cycle, for nappers and
split-sleepers.

$\phi = 17-25$ is virtually forbidden. (Section 4.3)

7. The distribution of sleep onsets is a bimodal function of circadian phase, with local maxima near low temperature $(\phi = 0)$ and nap phase $(\phi = 9-10)$. (Section 4.4.1)

8. The percent of time subjects are in bed varies almost sinusoidally with circadian phase. They are asleep about 50% of the time at $\phi = 3$, but only about 20% of the time near $\phi = 13-19$. (Section 4.4.2.1)

9. The rate of sleep onset depends on both circadian phase and prior wake length. The maximal rate is about 30% per hour, near $\phi = 2$ and $\phi = 10$. In other words, a wakeful subject has a 30% chance of falling asleep in the hour between $\phi = 2$ and $\phi = 3$. The minimal rate is about 6% per hour, at $\phi = 6$. Prolonged wakefulness increases the rate of sleep onset, moreso at some phases than at others. (Section 4.4.2.2)

10. (a) Few sleep onsets occur spontaneously in two "wake-maintenance zones." The morning zone is near $\phi = 5-7$, and the evening zone is near $\phi = 16-18$ (Section 4.5.1).

(b) In ultradian sleep studies, subjects slept least when put to bed in the evening zone (Section 4.5.2).

(c) On a constant routine, sleep-deprived subjects had the fewest microsleeps at 11 AM and midnight, times of day near the two zones (Section 4.5.3).

(d) A patient who was free-running in society, with bedtimes drifting uncontrollably around the clock, nevertheless selected the fewest bedtimes at hours corresponding to the zones (Section 4.5.4).

(e) Sleep onset insomnia was induced in a healthy subject by placing him on a 23.5h day, thereby drawing the evening zone later and locking it onto his scheduled bedtime (Section 4.5.5).

11. The period and phase of the pacemaker driving the temperature rhythm may be estimated from sleep data alone, using sleep onset clustering and sleep duration analyses. (Section 4.6)

12. The long-term behavior of the sleep-wake cycle remains mysterious. The hypothesis of secular lengthening holds less generally than once believed. (Section 4.8)

13. The period of the circadian temperature rhythm shortens by about 0.7h after internal synchrony is lost. (Section 4.9.1)

14. During internal synchrony there is a significant negative correlation between wake length and subsequent sleep length. On the other hand, sleep and following wake are uncorrelated. (Section 4.9.2)

15. For internally desynchronized subjects, the mean duration of wakefulness is practically independent of onset phase. Real data almost always disagree with model predictions here. (Section 4.9.3)

16 The relative predictability of sleep versus wake durations, given their respective onset phases, depends on the definition of "predictability". Compared to sleep, wake duration has a larger absolute uncertainty, but a smaller percent uncertainty, when a weighted average is taken across all onset phases. Yet in stark contrast to *sleep*, a knowledge of onset phase for *wake* cannot be used to improve the forecasted length of the episode (beyond that value expected from the overall mean.) (Section 4.9.3).

17. Subjects who nap or have split sleep episodes during free-run bear many resemblances to desynchronized subjects with long sleep-wake cycles: they exhibit circadian modulation of the timing and duration of sleep and wake. In particular, the phasing of wake- and sleep-maintenance zones agrees with that of desynchronized subjects. (Section 4.10)

Chapter 5

Theoretical Background

Internal desynchronization has stimulated a great deal of theorizing. Loosely speaking, most of the proposed models postulate one of two time-keeping mechanisms: a pair of self-sustained oscillators with continuous coupling (Sections 5.1–5.3) or a fatigue variable building up and decaying between circadian-modulated thresholds; (Sections 5.4–5.6). Other approaches are discussed in Section 5.7.

5.1 Conceptual Model of Aschoff and Wever

Aschoff and Wever (1976, 1981; Wever, 1975, 1979) offered an early understanding of internal desynchronization and man's circadian system in general. A circadian pacemaker was imagined to underlie the stable oscillation of core body temperature. Because the temperature rhythm persists in both period and amplitude, even in the absence of zeitgebers, they reasoned that the pacemaker is *self-sustained*, not damped or neutrally stable. Compared to temperature, the activity "rhythm" during desynchrony is much more variable, so much that one could question its intrinsic rhythmicity. As Aschoff (1965) wrote,

> The question whether both the frequencies... represent true circadian clocks is difficult to decide. It might be that we have to consider the unusual long behavioral periods as a kind of "artifact", while the primary clock system is reflected by the more nearly daily rhythms of body temperature and of excretion of water and potassium.

Nevertheless, Aschoff and Wever initiated a method of analysis that has become firmly entrenched: they ascribed a nominal period to the activity pattern by averaging the interval between successive wake-ups (or by running a regression line through mid-sleep.) Then, to explain this second "periodicity", Aschoff and Wever hypothesized that an independent, self-sustained pacemaker controls the sleep-wake alternation. Their reasoning: How could the rhythms of temperature and activity exhibit different overt periods if the same pacemaker were driving both? In their view two periods imply two clocks. Normally the two clocks interact so as to stay mutually synchronized, but their separate characters are revealed in desynchrony.

Furthermore, reasoned Aschoff and Wever, the clocks have different properties. After desynchronization, the temperature period shortens by much less than the activity period lengthens (Section 4.9.1) — hence the temperature pacemaker is "stronger" (in addition to being more "stable", as already mentioned). The pacemakers must be *mutually* coupled — since each changes its period away from the compromise enforced during synchrony — yet coupling is *almost unidirectional*, implying the temperature oscillator's relative "strength." The temperature pacemaker thus acts like an "internal zeitgeber".

5.2 Wever's Noninteractive Model

Wever (1975, 1979) has suggested a simple mathematical description of the two-oscillator concept. Temperature is principally controlled by a Type I oscillator, with some small "masking" contribution from the Type II oscillator dominating the activity cycle. Type I oscillators are "stronger" then Type II oscillators, and also more "stable", in the sense of less variability of period.

Wever's interesting point is that a mere *superposition* of such oscillations in many ways resembles the observed data. In other words, the outputs of the oscillators are summed but do not interact dynamically.

Let the Type I and II oscillations be represented as $X = \sin \omega_1 t$ and $Y = \sin(\omega_2 t + \phi)$, respectively. Then Wever's noninteractive model postulates that temperature T and activity A are convex linear combinations of X and Y:

$$A = aY + (1-a)X$$

$$T = bX + (1-b)Y.$$

Here $a > \frac{1}{2}$, $b > \frac{1}{2}$ so that T is dominated by X and A by Y. A threshold A_0 converts the continuous variable A to a discrete sleep-wake variable: sleep begins when A falls below A_0, and ends when A rises upward through A_0.

Wever's model suggests that beat phenomena with a period of a few cycles may underlie the "scalloping" patterns observed during desynchrony. The coincidence of sleep onsets with low temperature is commonly taken as evidence of a residual *coupling* between A and T, but Wever's model shows that scalloping arises even without any coupling whatsoever.

His model is mainly pedagogical — it warns us about the danger of inferences based on the superficial resemblance between data and simulated raster plots. (This is still the most frequent criterion by which models of free-run are judged.) When subjected to more discriminating tests, Wever's model fails (Section 7.3). Its main drawback is its fixed level threshold. Unrealistically long wake episodes occur during each beat cycle, when the amplitude of A becomes too small (Section 6.2).

5.3 Kronauer's XY Model: Coupled Van der Pol Oscillators

Kronauer and colleagues (1982, 1983, 1984) have developed a mathematical model of the human circadian system based on two coupled limit cycle oscillators. They have rendered precise many of Aschoff and Wever's qualitative concepts, and have extended those early ideas by introducing provocative accounts of spontaneous desynchrony (Kronauer *et al.*, 1982, 1983), entrainment to zeitgebers (Gander *et al.*, 1984a,b; Kronauer, 1984), sleep deprivation (Kronauer, 1983), and jet-lag (Gander *et al.*, 1985). Only the model of free-run will be considered in what follows.

Basic Properties of x and y

In Kronauer's model, "x" and "y" refer to two circadian pacemakers. They are analogous to the Type I and II oscillators of Wever (1975, 1979) (Figure 5-1) — x dominates the core body temperature rhythm, and y regulates the sleep-wake cycle. The pacemakers x and y are not to be regarded as synonymous with temperature and sleep; x and y are "clocks" which drive these overt rhythms, as well as several others (Moore-Ede $et\ al.$, 1982) such as urinary and hormone rhythms.

To account for the distinct frequencies observed during internal desynchronization, and the persistent amplitudes of the various circadian rhythms, x and y are postulated to be self-sustained oscillators (again following Aschoff and Wever). Specifically, they are assumed to be Van der Pol oscillators. This choice is motivated by mathematical simplicity: Van der Pol oscillators are analytically convenient and consequently there is a rich literature about them (Stoker, 1950; Minorsky, 1962). To rationalize phase-trapping, phase clustering, and the existence of a synchronized compromise period, the oscillators x and y are assumed to be mutually coupled. Because of relatively long-lived transients, such as those following release from entrainment, x and y are assumed to be only weakly nonlinear (i.e. their limit cycles are weakly attracting, rather than "stiff," like relaxation oscillators).

Equations and Parameter Estimation

The governing equations for free-running rhythms are

$$k^2\ddot{x} + k\mu_x(x^2-1)\dot{x} + (24/\hat{f}_x)^2 x + kF_{yx}\dot{y} = 0$$

$$k^2\ddot{y} + k\mu_y(y^2-1)\dot{y} + (24/\hat{f}_y)^2 y + kF_{xy}\dot{x} = 0$$

$\hat{f}_x, \hat{f}_y$ = intrinsic periods (in hours)

μ_x, μ_y = "stiffnesses" (dimensionless)

F_{yx}, F_{xy} = "impedances" or "coupling constants" (dimensionless)

$k = 24/2\pi$ (enables $\hat{f}$ to be expressed conveniently

in hours, instead of dimensionless "Kron-hours").

Kronauer $et\ al.$ (1982) estimate these parameters from the data, according to the following steps:

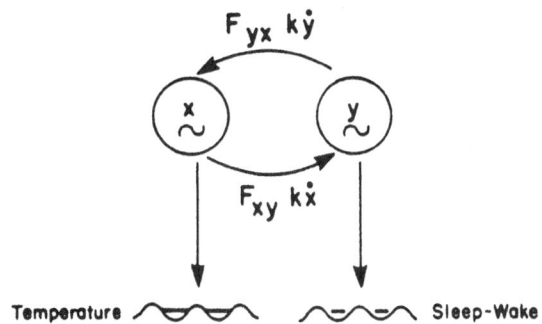

Oscillator x $\left[k^2\ddot{x}+k\mu_x(-1+x^2)\dot{x}+(24/\hat{\tau}_x)^2x\right]+F_{yx}k\dot{y}=0$

Oscillator y $\left[k^2\ddot{y}+k\mu_y(-1+y^2)\dot{y}+(24/\hat{\tau}_y)^2y\right]+F_{xy}k\dot{x}=0$

Figure 5-1. The XY model (Kronauer *et al.*, 1982, 1983) of the human circadian system, and the differential equations used to represent it. See text for definition of symbols. (Reproduced from Figure 4, Kronauer *et al.*, 1983).

(1) $\hat{f}_x$, $\hat{f}_y$ are near the observed periods of temperature and sleep observed at the *onset* of desynchrony.

(2) Estimates obtained in step (1) give F_{xy} via $|F_{xy}| = |\hat{\omega}_x - \hat{\omega}_y|$, where $\omega = 24/\tau$.

(3) The ratio F_{yx}/F_{xy} may be inferred from the observed compromise period and the results of step (1), as shown later for an analogous model [Section 6.3.5].

(4) F_{yx} is implied by steps (2) and (3).

(5) μ_y is inferred from the time course of phase adjustments after release from an entraining zeitgeber.

(6) μ_x is hard to extract, and is taken equal to μ_y.

As already mentioned, when estimated from real data, the stiffnesses μ are small (~ 0.1). Secondly the impedance ratio $F_{xy}/F_{yx} \sim 4/1$; thus x drives y strongly, yet is itself well-insulated from y's counter-influence. This corresponds to Aschoff and Wever's view of temperature as being controlled by a "strong," "Type I" oscillator.

Relations between x,y, Temperature and Sleep

Temperature as measured in the laboratory is a mixture of x (endogenous oscillation) and y ("evoked component," due to showers, exercise, changes in posture, etc.). In nearly all simulations to date, temperature is approximated by x alone.

Sleep has been treated in three ways in the XY model. The first version (Kronauer et al., 1982) assumes sleep to coincide with the central two-thirds of y's trough — with this selection, the "computer subject" sleeps about one-third of each cycle, independent of $\hat{f}_y$. The approach was abandoned because it requires the computer subject to foretell the future: it "cannot elect the time of sleep onset without knowing in advance when y will once again be positive" (Kronauer et al., 1983). The next version introduces two new variables, y_1, y_2 controlling separate ends of sleep. Sleep occurs when both y_1 and y_2 are below a zero threshold. Like the first criterion, the y_1, y_2 criteria essentially define sleep as occurring in a 120° wedge of y, $\dot{y}$ phase space (see Sections 6.2.3 and 6.4). Finally, because of a 2h phase inconsistency between the model and data (Kronauer et al., 1983), the most recent version shifts the y_1 and y_2 variables away from their symmetric position about minimum y; now y_2 marks the time when y crosses up through its mean, and y_1 lies about one-third of a cycle earlier (Gander et al., 1984a, 1985). Analytically, we have

$$y_1 = \alpha y - \dot{y}$$

$$y_2 = y$$

where $\alpha = -1/\sqrt{3} = -\cot(2\pi F)$, where $F = 1/3 =$ sleep fraction.

The Secular Drift of $\hat{\tau}_y$

One of the most interesting ideas in the original XY formulation (Kronauer *et al.*, 1982) is the postulate of a secularly increasing period $\hat{\tau}_y$. In simulations, when y's intrinsic period is allowed to lengthen gradually, the computer subject displays synchrony with internal phase drift, then phase-trapping, and then with apparent suddenness, internal desynchrony. All the qualitative phenomena of PR01 (Section 3.1) are reproduced in the proper sequence by the mere lengthening of a single parameter. Dramatically different phenomena are unified and explained by subtle internal changes.

No one understands why, physiologically speaking, $\hat{\tau}_y$ might lengthen. In any case, the evidence for a secular increase in $\hat{\tau}_y$ is weak (Section 4.8). Currently one is forced to say that $\hat{\tau}_y$ is "labile"; it can increase, decrease, oscillate with a $\sim$ 20-day period, etc. In a complete theory, $\hat{\tau}_y$ would itself be a dynamical variable. As matters stand, its time-evolution can be modeled only after the fact.

Concluding Remarks

(1) The importance of amplitude has been emphasized by Kronauer *et al.* (1982). Their limit cycle oscillators have amplitude as well as phase. Phase-trapping, in which x and y have the same average period, but their phase-relation varies periodically, is possible only in theories incorporating amplitude variables. For example, the gated pacemaker (Section 5.6) of Daan *et al.* (1984) corresponds to a stiff nonlinear oscillator and cannot phase-trap. For this reason, it is important to ascertain (Section 4.7) whether phase-trapping really is a prominent feature of human data.

(2) The x and y oscillators *mutually* interact. No one doubts that the temperature cycle strongly influences sleep; the question is, does y ("activity") feed back on x in any significant way? Daan *et al.* (1984) claim there is little evidence for such feedback. Kronauer and Gander (1984) again invoke phase-trapping, as well as the existence of a compromise period, as evidence for the y-drive onto x.

Furthermore, the XY model postulates that zeitgebers entrain x *only* through the influence of y. That is, zeitgebers act on y directly, which then mediates their influence on x. So Kronauer *et al.* (1982; Gander *et al.*, 1984a,b) see the $y \rightarrow x$ drive as crucial to the mechanism of entrainment. This interesting idea challenges the standard view of light-dark cycles acting directly on strong, stable circadian pacemakers (in this case, x).

(3) The anatomical structures corresponding to x and y is a matter of some controversy. The suprachiasmatic nuclei (SCN) in the mammalian hypothalamus are known to be circadian pacemakers (Moore-Ede *et al.*, 1982, Chapter 4). When the SCN are lesioned in primates (Fuller *et al.*, 1981), the activity rhythm vanishes but the temperature rhythm persists. A simple interpretation of this result (which is controversial) is that the SCN correspond to y, the "activity oscillator." Moreover, since the XY model postulates that y is the target of zeitgebers, it seems reasonable to identify y with the SCN: the SCN are believed to receive information about the light-dark cycle via inputs from the retinohypothalamic tract (Moore-Ede *et al.*, 1982, Chapter 4).

On the other hand, the y-oscillator may be more a mathematical construct or a behavioral descriptor than an anatomical entity. Its "period" as observed in the desynchronized sleep-wake cycle is "labile" and unpredictable. The y-oscillator shows an extremely wide range of entrainment. Winfree (1982b) has raised the possibility that activity, while strongly influenced by the circadian temperature pacemaker, is not intrinsically rhythmic. Indeed, what evidence is there for a y-rhythm at all? Physiological rhythms in the y-group (Moore-Ede et al., 1982) are arguably direct responses to sleep itself: slow-wave sleep is usually induced by the mere act of falling asleep, at any time of day; secretion of growth hormone is also triggered by sleep onset, and does not otherwise seem to be rhythmic; skin temperature of course depends directly on the state of activity. Therefore the evidence for a y-rhythm must, for the present, be sought in the patterns of sleep and wake alone.

For example, consider an experiment in which a desynchronized subject with $\hat{\tau}_y \sim 33h$ is suddenly placed on a "constant routine" (Czeisler et al., 1986) for 3 days. Would skin temperature, growth hormone, or any measure of activity display a 33h periodicity? Or would "clamping" sleep clamp these "rhythms" as well?

In contrast to y, the x-oscillator is stable and robust in the way that circadian pacemakers usually are. It may correspond to the SCN, as further suggested by melatonin data. Melatonin is secreted by the pineal, which is regulated by a circadian rhythm of neural impulses from the SCN (Lewy, 1983). Lewy and Newsome (1983) report the case of a blind person whose activity/rest cycle was normally entrained but whose melatonin secretory maximum delayed by 4-6h each successive week for 4 weeks. In other words, his melatonin rhythm was free-running. Their preliminary evidence suggests that "the melatonin rhythm and the temperature rhythm are phase-locked in these blind subjects, which implies that they are controlled by the same endogenous pacemaker" (Lewy, 1983). The implied logic is that the SCN regulates the pineal, and the output of the pineal is phase-locked with temperature — hence the SCN may also drive the endogenous temperature cycle, thus identifying the SCN with x.

(4) The preceding discussion about the anatomical basis of y raises the question most likely to agitate a circadian modeler: what is an oscillator, and in particular, is the sleep-wake alternation controlled by one? Some people (usually mathematicians) use the words "rhythm" and "oscillation" interchangeably — both refer to a time-varying process which repeats itself. In this view, if an oscillation is present, then so is an oscillator. Hence the sleep-wake alternation is (trivially) controlled by an oscillator. Moreover since all models of internal desynchronization generate two periodicities, they are all two-oscillator models. (For examples of this sort of argument, see Kronauer and Gander (1984), or the discussion following the Eastman (1984) and Daan and Beersma (1984) papers.)

The other side (usually biologists) reply that some oscillations are driven by pacemakers, and others are not. Rhythm generators for breathing or the heartbeat are the prototypical pacemakers to be kept in mind: not mathematical constructs but warm, biological, anatomically based entities that produce regular oscillations in voltages, hormone levels, or other experimentally measurable quantities. This definition sometimes includes period regulation — some restorative mechanism opposes deviation away from a standard period. In this view, the relaxation oscillatory S process (Section 5.6) of Daan et al. (1984) is not a pacemaker because transient elevations of the sleep onset threshold would lengthen both sleep and wake, producing a positive correlation between the two halves of the cycle, rather than the negative correlation some require in a "pacemaker." This is why many biologists feel that the Daan model involves only one circadian pacemaker.

For the record, my feeling is that all models of desynchrony involve two oscillators, but that the sleep-wake cycle is probably not controlled by a circadian pacemaker.

5.4 Conceptual Model of Borbély

Borbély (1982) has proposed a model of sleep regulation which unifies findings from classical sleep research with those of the more recent circadian studies. His model has intuitive and physiological appeal, and it has inspired the quantitative work of Daan and Beersma (Daan and Beersma, 1984; Daan et al., 1984; and see Section 5.6).

Processes S and C

In Borbely's model, sleep is regulated by two processes, S and C. The S variable corresponds loosely to "fatigue," and may actually represent a neurochemical sleep promoting factor (reviewed by Borbély and Tobler, 1980). It builds up during waking hours and decays during sleep. However, studies of prolonged sleep deprivation (Akerstedt and Froberg, 1977; Gulevich et al., 1966) have shown that fatigue does not increase monotonically with waking time, but rather oscillates with a marked circadian rhythm. Thus Borbély also postulated the C process, a circadian component of sleep regulation. C is taken to be independent of earlier sleeping or waking.

The sum of S and C represents the total sleep propensity. A sleep episode ends when this sum falls below a certain threshold. A convenient way to visualize this is shown in Figure 5-2. The modulated threshold $\overline{C}$ is the negative of C; now wake-up occurs when S falls below $\overline{C}$.

Exponential Decay of S

One key point of the Borbely model is that S decays exponentially during sleep. The assumption is based on two facts: (1) Borbély's electrophysiological measurements indicate that the integrated EEG power density in the low frequency range (roughly speaking, slow-wave activity) decays exponentially during a sleep episode (Borbély et al., 1981). Here slow-waves are taken as the EEG correlate of process S, a reasonable assumption since slow-wave sleep is known to depend on prior waking (reviewed in Borbély, 1982). For example, there is a massive increase in the initial level of slow-wave activity after prolonged sleep deprivation. (2) It is well known that sleep duration does *not* increase linearly with prior waking. After a world record performance of 264h of continuous wakefulness, (some of it spent playing games in a penny arcade), a subject slept for only 14.4h (Gulevich et al., 1966). Thus even if process S builds up to enormous levels, if it is dissipated exponentially fast the subsequent sleep will not be excessively long.

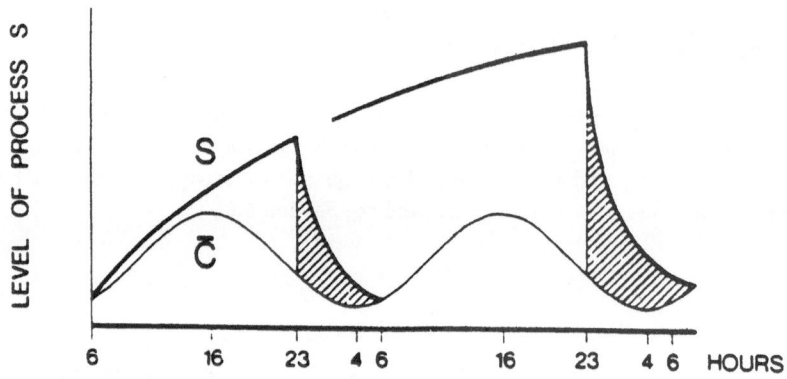

Figure 5-2. Timecourse of Process S and the negative function of Process C (curve $\bar{C}$, in the model of Borbély(1982). Sleep occurs during the shaded regions and ends when S falls below $\bar{C}$. The timecourse of Process S during sleep following a regular waking period (left) is compared to its timecourse after a period of sleep deprivation (right). (Reproduced from Figure 4, Borbély, 1982).

Temperature, Process C, and Sleep Duration

The circadian threshold $\overline{C}$ is assumed sinusoidal and in phase with the circadian temperature cycle. This choice incorporates the established relation between rhythms of alertness and temperature (Czeisler *et al*, 1980a; Colquhoun, 1971). Moreover, it predicts qualitatively the relation between sleep duration and circadian phase of sleep onset (Section 4.1.1). Borbély compared his model to the sleep deprivation data of Akerstedt and Gillberg (1981), and showed that increasing wakefulness was followed by *shorter* sleep, but only up to a point. After that, sleep duration increases dramatically and then proceeds to shorten again. In Borbély's model, the jump in duration occurs for sleep begun slightly after the maximum of $\overline{C}$ — in fact, an earlier phase is indicated by the data (Section 4.1.1). Nevertheless the qualitative agreement is revealing because it indicates how easily a modulated threshold model can account for the sleep duration data.

Concluding Remarks

(1) Borbély's (1982) model focuses on sleep regulation but postulates no complementary mechanisms for wake regulation. Thus his model addresses half of the sleep-wake cycle. Daan *et al*. (1984) completed the picture by proposing a *second* circadian-modulated threshold: it determines the time of sleep onset. This more elaborate model is discussed in Section 5.6.

(2) Borbely's identification of an exponentially declining process S with slow-wave activity implies that the end of a long sleep episode should contain very little slow-wave sleep. The model may need to be amended in this regard — as Borbély himself admits, a "peculiar feature that was occasionally observed for very long sleep periods consisted in a second SWS [slow-wave sleep] peak 12-18h after sleep onset (Webb, 1978b; Weitzman *et al*, 1979)." (See Section 3.7 for an example.)

Moreover, Gagnon and DeKoninck (1981, 1982) have found similar reappearances of slow-wave sleep in subjects who managed to voluntarily extend their wake-up time for several hours. (This overriding of the wake-up threshold in itself poses problems for Borbély's model!) One type of slow-wave bout appeared in the afternoon nap phase, independent of the time of sleep onset. This may reflect an unsuspected circadian influence on slow-wave sleep. The other anomalous slow-wave activity occurred 12h after sleep onset, as found by the authors above.

(3) The internal organization of sleep in terms of REM and the stages of non-REM sleep is almost never considered in models of the sleep-wake cycle. Borbély (1982) was one of the first to do so. Consistent with the literature showing that the amount of REM sleep is less influenced by prior sleep-wake history than by the circadian temperature cycle, Borbély (1982) postulated that REM reflects the level of process C. Slow-wave sleep is of course linked to process S and does depend strongly on prior sleeping and waking. The REM/non-REM cycle is treated as in McCarley and Hobson (1975) but with parameters modulated by the circadian process C. Theories about how the circadian cycle interacts with the REM/non-REM cycle offer intriguing possibilities for future research (McCarley and Massaquoi, 1983).

5.5 Winfree's Half-model

Winfree (1983, 1984) has emphasized an asymmetry in the free-running human sleep-wake cycle: though the duration of a sleep episode depends predictably on the circadian phase of sleep onset (Section 4.1.1), no comparable regularity has ever been found which predicts the duration of subsequent wakefulness, given prior events. For example the phase of wake-up, or the length of the prior sleep, each fail to predict the length of the following wake episode (Section 4.9.3). This asymmetry between the timing of sleep and wake "impugns the reliability of models that treat sleep onset and wake onset as complementary but comparable processes" (Winfree, 1983); many of the models discussed in this chapter do exactly that. Winfree alone seems to have recognized this drawback. To offer one of many examples, the symmetrical treatment of sleep and wake onset in Kronauer's model (Section 5.3) gives rise to an unrealistically precise relation between wake duration and the phase of wake-up. In Section 7.4.6, the wake duration data are used to test each of the models considered there.

Because of his avowed "inability to make sense of wake duration data," Winfree (1983) has attempted to model only the sleep half of the sleep-wake cycle. He developed the model originally to account for the circadian gating of eclosion in *Drosophila* (Winfree, 1980) but he reinterprets it to account for the circadian gating of wake-up in humans (Winfree, 1983; 1984).

The model resembles Borbély's (1982): "restedness" accumulates during sleep until it crosses a threshold, at which time wake-up occurs. Restedness is assumed to equal the cumulative sleep time, and so increases linearly in time. The threshold is rhythmically modulated, either by an environmental zeitgeber, or by an endogenous circadian clock, if zeitgebers are absent. (Figure 5-3).

The threshold oscillations do not necessarily correspond to any physiological observable, though Winfree (1983) notes that free-running humans behave as if the threshold oscillation and the core body temperature oscillation were in phase.

Winfree's work (1983; 1984) differs from Borbély's (1982) mainly in emphasis: Winfree makes less attempt to relate his model to sleep stages and focuses instead on its mathematical properties. His main points concern the model's predictions about wake-up timing and sleep duration, and the dependence of those predictions on the parameters in the model. When the modulation amplitude is sufficiently strong, sleep duration becomes a discontinuous function of phase of sleep onset, with a jump between the longest and shortest sleeps beginning at nearly the same phase. Such a jump is typical of real data (Section 4.1.1). In the model, this jump is due to restedness either just grazing the threshold, or else slipping past to produce a long sleep (Figure 5-3). As Winfree points out, a jump in the sleep duration curve translates to a gap in the phases of wake-up, a "forbidden zone" for spontaneous waking (see Section 4.3). When the modulation amplitude is smaller than a critical amount, the gap in the wake-up phases disappears, though there is still a tendency for those phases to be sampled less frequently than others at which the threshold is being hit broadside.

The upshot is that modulated-threshold models produce different dependences of sleep duration on sleep onset phase, according the amplitude of threshold modulation. As amplitude goes from zero to large values, the sleep duration curve goes from flat, to unimodal, to skewed with a steep upslope, to a ramp with an outright discontinuity (Figure 5-4). The

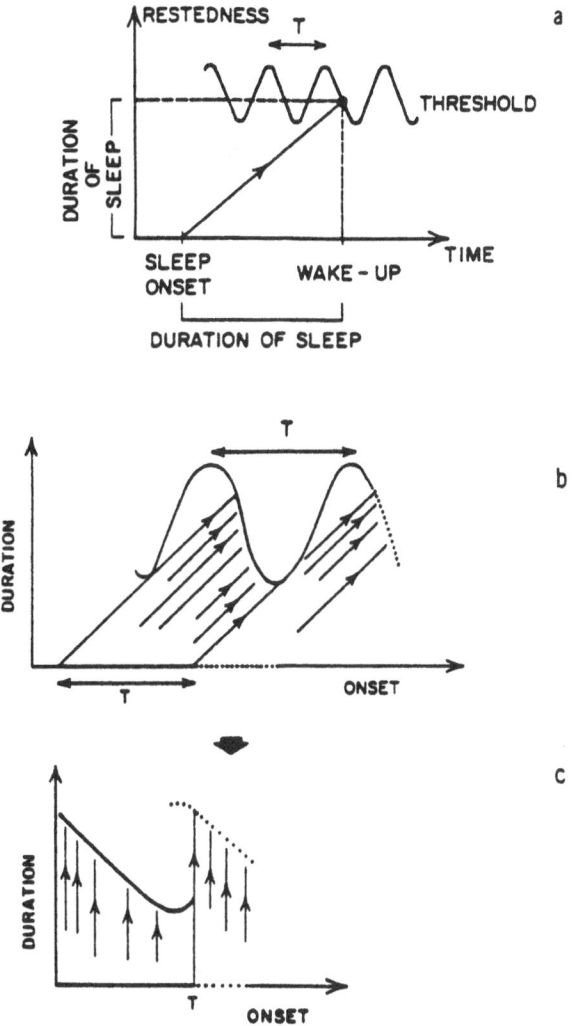

Figure 5-3

(a) In the model of Winfree (1983), restedness is assumed proportional to cumulative sleep. It rises toward a wake-up threshold which is modulated by a circadian rhythm. One particular choice of sleep onset time is shown.

(b) As in (a), but with threshold interceptions occurring over a range of sleep onset phases.

(c) The dependence of sleep duration on choice of sleep onset phase, as implied by (b). A jump in sleep duration occurs at the critical sleep onset phase from which restedness rises to a *tangent* intersection with the threshold.

(Reproduced from Figures 3, 4 of Winfree, 1984).

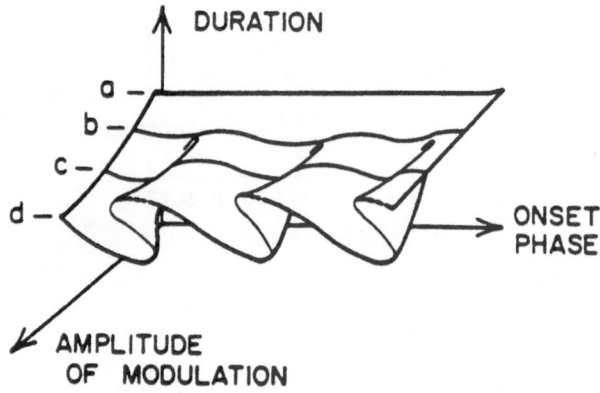

Figure 5-4. Models with modulated thresholds produce different $\phi_s:\rho$ relationships (Section 4.1.1), depending on the amplitude of the circadian modulation.
With no modulation (a), duration is independent of phase. Slight modulation
(b) yields a sinusoidal $\phi_s:\rho$ curve. As modulation increases the curve
develops a steep upslope (c), and ultimately a discontinuity (d). Sleep length
is double-valued near this discontinuity.

(Reproduced from Figure 7, Winfree, 1984)

dependence of sleep duration on its two control parameters — sleep onset phase and amplitude modulation — is thus seen to be structured by a "cusp catastrophe" (Zeeman, 1977).

5.6 Gated Pacemaker of Daan, Beersma, and Borbély

Summary of the Model

The conceptual model of Borbély (1982) has been formalized and extended by Daan and Beersma (1984). In this model and its further elaboration (Daan *et al.*, 1984), two processes called S and C regulate the sleep-wake cycle. Process S builds up during wakefulness and decays during sleep, precisely as in Borbély's (1982) model. Sleep onset occurs when S crosses a high threshold H, and wake-up occurs when S falls below a low threshold L (Figure 5-5).

Process C is generated by a single circadian pacemaker and it imposes an approximately sinusoidal modulation on the thresholds. Hence there are circadian influences on the sleep-wake fluctuations: Process C strongly synchronizes S if the threshold oscillations have large amplitude A; otherwise S adopts a periodicity governed mainly by the separation of the thresholds H and L.

Finally, to model the observed variability in sleep-wake data, and to prevent the system from locking into an unrealistically precise synchrony, subharmonic or otherwise, Daan *et al.* (1984) postulate that the thresholds H and L are slightly noisy. Zero-mean Gaussian random variables are resampled and added to the threshold mean levels $\bar{H}$ and $\bar{L}$ at each time step in computer simulations of the model. The levels of noise are chosen to match Wever's (1979) results on the correlation structure of the sleep-wake cycle during internal synchrony.

Model Interpretation of Sleep-Wake Manipulations

Before presenting the details of the model, it is instructive to consider qualitatively how it may be used to simulate a range of phenomena. (Chapter 7 quantitatively compares the model's simulations to free-run data.)

Entrainment: Process C is synchronized to the 24h cycle, and the threshold modulation amplitude is large, reflecting a "resonance" with external zeitgebers. Thus the model predicts that S also becomes entrained, with a characteristic phase relation to C that depends on the choice of model parameters.

Free-run: In the absence of zeitgebers, the modulation amplitude A is assumed to decrease, and process C adopts its natural period τ. S remains synchronized to C unless A is too small, in which case S desynchronizes. Thus the model ascribes internal desynchrony to a reduction in the circadian modulation amplitude.

Sleep Deprivation: To a large extent Borbély's (1982) model was designed to account for sleep deprivation data. This inherent feature of the model is retained in the mathematical version of Daan *et al.* (1984). For example, to simulate the effects of enforced wakefulness, the upper threshold H is assumed inoperative (or equivalently, H is set equal to the upper asymptote for the exponential S process). Hence S is allowed to attain unusually high levels, which would account for the enhanced slow-wave activity after sleep deprivation.

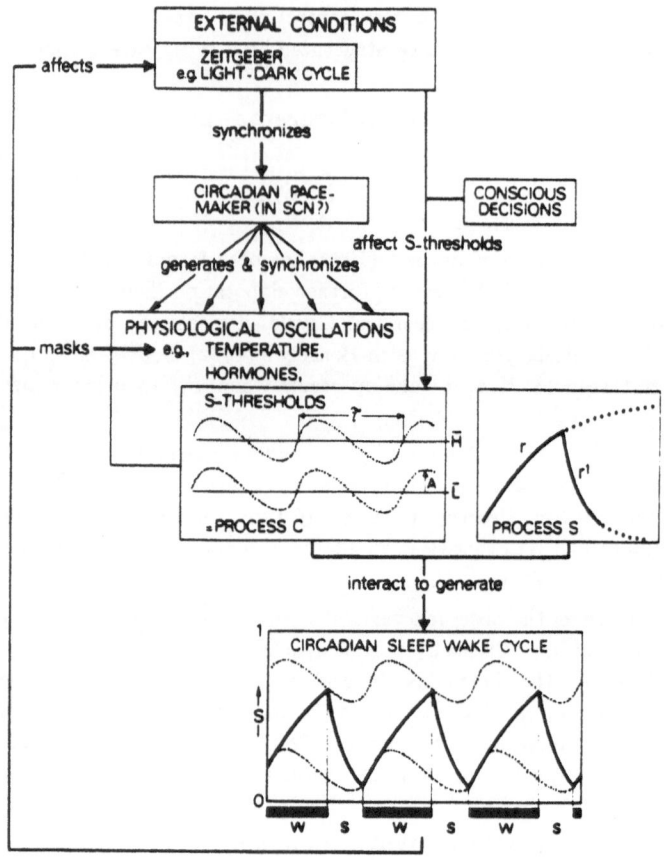

Figure 5-5. The gated pacemaker of Daan, Beersma, and Borbély (1984). See text for explanation of symbols.

(Reproduced from Figure 1, Daan *et al.* (1984).)

When recovery sleep begins, S drops rapidly from its elevated value. The data of Akerstedt and Gillberg (1981) on the duration of recovery sleep after variable amounts of sleep deprivation have been used to estimate the precise shape of the lower threshold L (Daan et al., 1984). Thus sleep deprivation data are built into the model in at least two ways: they are used to determine the rising S kinetics during wakefulness, and to specify the shape of the wake-up threshold L. Finally, the distance between S and L can be taken as a measure of sleep propensity (as in Borbély, 1982). During prolonged wakefulness, this measure increases exponentially but it is modulated by a circadian rhythm, a result observed in empirical studies (Akerstedt and Froberg, 1977).

Continuous Bedrest: Daan et al. (1984) make much of Campbell's (1984) data on continuous bedrest. In these experiments, subjects were told to lie quietly for 60 hours and were isolated from time cues and stimulation. Exercise, reading, listening to music, etc. were forbidden. They were allowed to turn a 60 watt tablelamp on and off as they wished — it was the only source of illumination. In this constant "disentrained" environment the subjects' sleep-wake patterns fragmented, with a mean sleep-wake cycle length of 6.1h and a mean sleep fraction of 48% (Campbell, 1984). In spite of the polyphasic sleep pattern, there was a persistent circadian oscillation in sleep duration, with the greatest sleep length (mean = 6.3h) for episodes begun between 24:00h and 01:00h.

To simulate the effects of continuous bedrest, Daan et al. (1984) suggest that $\bar{H}$ be lowered dramatically. This corresponds to the common-sense expectation that in the boring environment of Campbell's experiment, the subjects had a lowered threshold for falling asleep (since there was little else to do!). With the appropriate choice of $\bar{H}$, the simulation results are reported to match the data on average sleep fraction and sleep-wake cycle length. The interesting point here is that with *one* free parameter $(\bar{H})$, *two* features of data seem to be encompassed. In contrast, the XY model (Section 5.3) would need a change in the values of two parameters — sleep fraction and $\hat{r}_y$ — to account for Campbell's data.

One caveat: Longer bedrest studies (Ohta et al., 1983) have found large sleep fractions only in the first two days of the experiment, with a return to $\sim 30\%$ after three days, suggesting that Campbell's results may represent transient phenomena.

Parameter Estimation

Daan et al. (1984) have estimated the rise and decay rates of S from the EEG data of Borbély et al. (1981). If the upper and lower asymptotes for S are scaled to be 0 and 1, then the assumed kinetics are:

$$S_i = 0.888 \, S_{i-1} \qquad \text{(decay during sleep)}$$

$$S_i = 1 - 0.973 \, (1-S_{i-1}) \quad \text{(rise during wake)}$$

where the time step is one half hour. Converted to half-life time constants, the two rates correspond to ~ 13h (wake) and ~ 3h (sleep). This asymmetry of rates, in which the S process decays four times more rapidly than it builds up, is an essential asymmetry in the model.

As already mentioned, the noise in the thresholds is chosen to match Wever's (1979) correlation data for synchronized free-run. At each time-step in the computer simulations, a variable $y_i = \tfrac{1}{2}y_{i-1} + x$ is added to both thresholds. The random variable x is normally distributed with zero mean and standard deviation $p = 0.022$.

The lower threshold L is derived from Akerstedt and Gillberg's (1981) data on the duration of recovery sleep after sleep deprivation. The result is a skewed sine wave with a fast rise and slow decay.

The upper threshold H is problematic for the model. It is regarded as highly dependent on environmental conditions and subjective factors. Dark rooms, boring lectures, bedrest and hot afternoons tend to lower H, while lively conversations and good books tend to raise it. In the absence of contradictory information, and to keep the number of free parameters to a minimum, Daan *et al.* (1984) have assumed that H has the same amplitude and phase as L, but is displaced upward from it.

The mean levels $\bar{H}$ and $\bar{L}$ of the thresholds determine the approximate sleep fraction and sleep-wake periodicity (if the modulation A were zero, $\bar{H}$ and $\bar{L}$ would determine them *exactly* — see Section 6.5.2). Depending on the conditions — entrainment, free-run, continuous bedrest, etc. — only a narrow range of $\bar{H}$ and $\bar{L}$ are possible. Quantitative exploration of the $H-L$ parameter space is the topic of Section 6.5.2.

Concluding Remarks

(1) The model of Daan *et al.* (1984) assumes a direct chain of control: zeitgebers synchronize the circadian pacemaker, which in turn modulates the sleep-wake cycle through the thresholds for process S. Several questions are left unanswered. How do zeitgeters influence C? Daan *et al.* (1984) refer to a possible mechanism based on a phase-response curve to light, but its details are deliberately left unspecified until experimental data are available. Yet much entrainment data is *already* available — Wever (1979) presents a number of studies which constrain the possible mechanisms. Kronauer, Gander and coworkers have taken on the challenge of Wever's data, with some encouraging results (Gander *et al.*, 1984a,b; Kronauer, 1984).

5.7 Other Approaches

This section reviews a number of mathematical models of circadian rhythms which, while deserving attention, will not be analyzed extensively in subsequent chapters. Some of the models address human sleep-wake rhythms (Dirlich, 1984; Eastman, 1984) but it is unclear how to test them. Others are concerned less with the details of human rhythms, and more with mammalian rhythms (Daan and Berde, 1978; Carpenter and Grossberg, 1983, 1984) or even more general classes of circadian rhythms (Wever, 1984b; Enright, 1980).

5.7.1 Phase-shift models

These models (Kawato *et al.*, 1982; Eastman, 1984; Daan and Berde, 1978) are related by their shared use of phase-response curves, a concept which has dominated the theoretical analysis of biological rhythms (Pavlidis, 1973; Pittendrigh, 1981; Moore-Ede *et al.*, 1982).

Model of Kawato *et al.*

Kawato *et al.* (1982) denote their attention to internal desynchronization in humans, especially to the phenomenon of "forbidden wake-up" (Section 4.3; Winfree, 1982a). They consider a three-oscillator model composed of simple clocks (Winfree, 1980) i.e. phase-only oscillators, which separately control temperature, sleep onset, and wake-up. The key assumption is that at a certain phase in the temperature cycle, the temperature oscillator emits a pulse stimulus to the sleep onset oscillator, resetting it via a phase response curve. Because of a coupling mechanism, the phase of wake-up is also reset. The form of the phase response curve is derived from the sleep duration data of Zulley *et al.* (1981). To be at all realistic the model requires three oscillators; with only two, the authors show that certain discontinuities are incorrectly predicted to exist in the sleep duration data.

Eastman's model

Eastman (1984) asks a provocative question in the title of her article "Are separate temperature and activity oscillators necessary to explain the phenomena of human circadian rhythms?" Her answer is "no," and she proposes a model of internal desynchronization involving entities like consciousness and voluntary behavior, masking and sleep need, instead of an activity oscillator. (See Section 5.3, Concluding Remark #4 for the one- vs. two-oscillator debate.) In Eastman's model, a circadian pacemaker drives the temperature rhythm at a period which may be observed directly only during internal synchronization; when the subject desynchronizes, the "misplaced" sleep episodes are assumed to cause small phase advances to the temperature cycle, perhaps because of light perceived upon awakening. With this feedback from activity to the pacemaker, Eastman's model can account for the shortening of the temperature period observed after desynchronization (Section 4.9.1). Note that in this model, the "intrinsic circadian period" is manifested only during synchrony and measurements of the period during desynchrony are regarded as contaminated — exactly opposite to the view of Kronauer *et al.* (1982).

The problem with the Eastman model is that it is not predictive with respect to the sleep-wake cycle, nor does it attempt to be, as was made plain in the following interchange between Czeisler and Eastman (p. 102, Moore-Ede and Czeisler, 1984):

Dr. Czeisler: When you model these shifts [of sleep-wake timing], do you have to take the original data, program each shift into a computer, and then say, "Now, there is another shift"? If so, it would then become a question of whether you have a model or whether you are just telling the computer to reproduce the actual data.

Dr. Eastman: Well, the model predicts that the subject will usually go to sleep on the minimum [of temperature], and it will soon, I hope, predict how much feedback there is.

Of course, if the subject skips the minimum because of some reason that only he knows (for example, if he is reading a book), we could never hope to predict that. So, of course, I have to copy that from the real data.

Enright (1984) also suggested the existence of cognitive interactions with the protocol as a cause of desynchrony, and like Eastman (1984), Enright emphasized the possible phase-shifting of the pacemaker by self-administered light stimuli. Apparently exasperated by the use of such unquantifiable notions as "cognitive interactions," Czeisler (p. 208, Moore-Ede and Czeisler, 1984) tartly replied to Enright that "the people who have not done actual experiments on human subjects .... are most concerned about the volitional aspect...". (Also, see Section 4.9.3 for further discussion of this controversial point.)

5.7.2 Models of Circadian Rhythms in General

Stochastic models

Dirlich (1984) and Enright (1980) address the question of the precision of circadian rhythms. In each case a large network of sloppy oscillators is shown to be capable of generating precise oscillations, thanks to coupling interactions among the elemental oscillators. Both authors emphasize the stochastic character of biological oscillations. But whereas Enright (1980) is careful to compare his model to biological data from a number of species, Dirlich (1984) explores a formal complex system to provoke the development of new circadian models.

Model of Carpenter and Grossberg

Carpenter and Grossberg (1983, 1984) propose a neural model for the mammalian SCN pacemaker. The model is used to simulate Aschoff's rule, the circadian rule, splitting, aftereffects, and phase-response curves.

The model consists of processes with direct physiologic interpretations: on-cells and off-cells; feedback signals via slowly accumulating transmitter substances; an ultradian fatigue process; and a slow gain process with a time scale of months. One drawback of any model which attempts such realism is the unavoidably large number of adjustable parameters and functional forms.

Model of Daan and Berde

Daan and Berde (1978) are also concerned with splitting, aftereffects and Aschoff's rule, but their approach is opposite to that of Carpenter and Grossberg; they construct an extremely simple but abstract model; "using it more to display and organize consequences of a general two-oscillator scheme than to yield mechanistic predictions." The model consists of a morning and evening activity oscillator, defined only in terms of their periods, phases, and mutually induced phase shifts. In particular, the oscillations have no amplitude variables. Their model is the difference equation analog of the differential equation PHASE model presented in Section 6.3.

Wever's Van der Pol model

Wever (1984b) summarizes his previous extensive research on nonlinear oscillator models of circadian rhythms. The equations discussed include both single and multiple oscillators. Wever feels it necessary to introduce awkward nonlinearities in his equations to prevent certain variables from ever going negative (the rationale offered is that certain biological variables must be positive, and hence so must the corresponding state variable in the equations). Unfortunately the resulting equations are hard to analyze. Two coupled nonlinear equations are used to generate waveforms representing activity and temperature. A flat threshold is applied to the activity rhythm to produce a discrete sleep-wake alternation, as in the noninteractive model of Section 5.2.

Chapter 6

Analysis of Models

6.1 Introduction

This chapter explores the mathematical structure of models of the sleep-wake cycle. As in other chapters, we focus on the empirical phenomenon of spontaneous internal desynchronization between the sleep-wake and temperature cycles during free-run. Other important phenomena such as those occurring during sleep deprivation, continuous bedrest or entrainment to 24h or other schedules, will not be discussed. As we shall see, understanding and accounting for internal desynchronization alone is a difficult task.

A parsimonious explanation of desynchrony based on a two-oscillator model has been offered by Kronauer *et al.* (1982, 1983), and was reviewed in Section 5.3. In that model, the y waveform governing the timing of sleep and wake is actually a sum of *two* components: The intrinsic y component and a significant circadian component due to coupling to the x oscillator. The explanation of spontaneous desynchronization is based on a hypothesized spontaneous lengthening of $\hat{r}_y$. As the disparity between $\hat{r}_x$ and $\hat{r}_y$ increases, x exerts less and less influence on the output of y. As Kronauer *et al.* (1983, p. 183) explain

> Clearly there is a dramatic change in the timing of sleep when desynchrony occurs yet there is only a very small change in the y waveform. This is the crucial lesson given by the model. In mathematical terms the distinction between phase-trapping and desynchrony is that in phase-trapping the "x component of y" is larger than the "intrinsic component of y" while in desynchrony it is the intrinsic component which is larger.

In other words, desynchrony is viewed by Kronauer *et al.* as a *beat phenomenon*, based on the summation of two waveforms to generate an admixture.

To expose the implications of the beat mechanism in their most transparent form, a model called BEATS is introduced in Section 6.2. It is a modification of an idea in Wever (1979), and its mathematical structure can be understood more easily than the coupled non-linear oscillator of Kronauer *et al.*

An issue raised by the BEATS model involves the conversion of a continuous waveform $y(t)$ into a discrete sleep-wake process. This conversion is ordinarily effected by thresholds: in Wever (1979), sleep occurs when $y(t)$ falls below a certain *level threshold*. Kronauer *et al.* (1982, 1983) criticized this approach and replaced it with an *angular threshold*, which depends less on the amplitude of y. With an angular threshold, sleep occurs when the smoothly varying y process enters a certain angular sector or wedge of state space.

The model of Daan *et al.* (1984) also involves thresholds in a central way. They postulate a pair of thresholds H and L controlling sleep onset and wake-up, respectively. When the S process reaches one of these thresholds, a change in kinetics is instantly triggered, and S moves toward the other threshold.

Through the simple BEATS model, we can better understand the formal relation between the models of Kronauer *et al.* and Daan *et al.* The phase plane analysis of all three models is a central theme in this chapter.

Another set of questions concerns the role of waveform "amplitude" in model structure. In the *XY* model of Kronauer *et al.*, a desynchronized sleep-wake cycle occurs when the *y* amplitude falls (due to a near cancellation of the intrinsic and *x* components of *y*), and the *y* process skips a threshold crossing. But how essential is this mechanism to the occurrence of desynchrony?

To explore the role of amplitude, a model of two coupled oscillators with *unchanging* amplitude is developed in Section 6.3. This model is called PHASE because it assumes that there are two pacemakers, one for sleep-wake and one for temperature, and that these are *phase-only oscillators*. That is, each has a one-dimensional circular state space. In this model, the notions of angular and level thresholds coincide; sleep occurs on a certain arc of one of the circles. PHASE is the simple differential equation model of two coupled self-sustained oscillators. It requires four parameters: two intrinsic periods and two coupling coefficients. Exact analytical solutions are possible for certain versions of the model. PHASE can be regarded as a stripped-down version of the XY model. It retains the essential ideas of coupling and self-sustainment of nonlinear oscillators. However phase-trapping is lost, because it requires an amplitude variable. In this respect, PHASE is closer to the Daan model than to the XY or BEATS models.

Overview

The chapter begins with the BEATS and PHASE models. Their properties are explored graphically and analytically. The XY model is studied next and connections are made to the simpler models. Finally, the Daan model is presented and an important oversight about the choice of its parameters is discussed. Phase plane analysis is used to interrelate all four models.

6.2 BEATS Model

6.2.1 Introduction

In Section 5.2 we considered Wever's noninteractive model of the sleep-wake cycle and the temperature rhythm. Both rhythms are regarded as superpositions of two sinusoidal oscillations, *X* and *Y*, with temperature dominated by *X* and activity by *Y*.

This section addresses the original model as well as two variants which use different threshold criteria to define when sleep occurs. One of these variants resembles the *XY* model of Kronauer *et al.* (Section 5.3) while the other behaves qualitatively like the gated pacemaker of Daan *et al.* (Section 5.6). Thus a simple model offers a unified view of two more complex models and shows precisely how they differ.

The family of models based on sums of sine waves will henceforth be called BEATS, because of the prominent role that beat phenomena play in the simulations, e.g. "scalloping" of the activity rhythm during internal desynchronization.

6.2.2 Rhythms

It is convenient to choose the unit of time such that the frequency of the circadian rhythm X is unity. In these units the frequency of Y is denoted ω; normally

$$\omega \leq 1 \ ,$$

i.e. the activity rhythm has longer period than the circadian oscillation. The equations for X and Y are chosen to be:

$$X = -\cos t \tag{6.1}$$

$$Y = -\cos(\omega t + \gamma) \tag{6.2}$$

This choice may look unnatural, but notice that it places the minimum of X at $t = 0$. This convention agrees with that of earlier chapters in which the educed temperature rhythm was used as a marker of circadian phase ϕ, with $\phi = 0$ along the midline of a raster plotted at the circadian period. In the simulations of BEATS, the locus $\phi = 0$ is automatically along the midline of the normalized raster because of the convention in (6.1).

Now the activity-rest rhythm A and the temperature rhythm T are modeled as superpositions of X and Y:

$$A = aY + (1-a)X \tag{6.3}$$

$$T = bX + (1-b)Y \tag{6.4}$$

where $a, b \in [0,1]$. The model rhythms are summarized in Figure 6-1.

6.2.3 Thresholds for Sleep and Wake

Level Threshold

In the model described by Wever (1979, p. 229), sleep is taken to occur when $A < A_0$, where A_0 is called a *level threshold* (distinguished from the angular threshold discussed later). Downward crossing of the threshold triggers sleep, and upward crossing of the same threshold awakens the (computer) subject (Figure 6-2). Note that one should intuitively equate A with "activity" or "alertness" rather than "sleepiness", since activity occurs when A is high (the convention is similar to Kronauer (1982) but *opposite* from Daan (1984).

The main problem with the level threshold criterion is that it produces unrealistically long wake episodes during internal desynchronization. They arise from "beats," in which

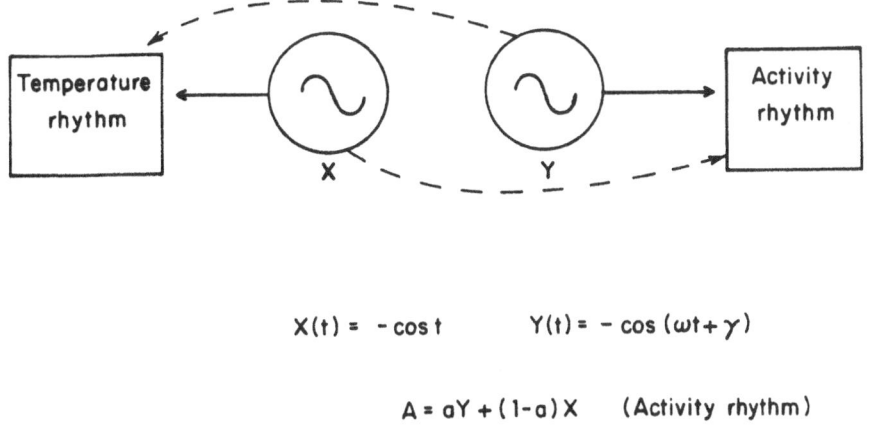

BEATS model structure
(based on Wever, 1979)

$$X(t) = -\cos t \qquad Y(t) = -\cos(\omega t + \gamma)$$

$$A = aY + (1-a)X \qquad \text{(Activity rhythm)}$$
$$T = bX + (1-b)Y \qquad \text{(Temperature rhythm)}$$

Figure 6-1. BEATS model of circadian rhythms of activity (A) and temperature (T). Pacemakers X and Y generate rhythms which are then added in different proportions to form A and T. A is dominated by Y and T is dominated by X. No coupling is assumed between X and Y.

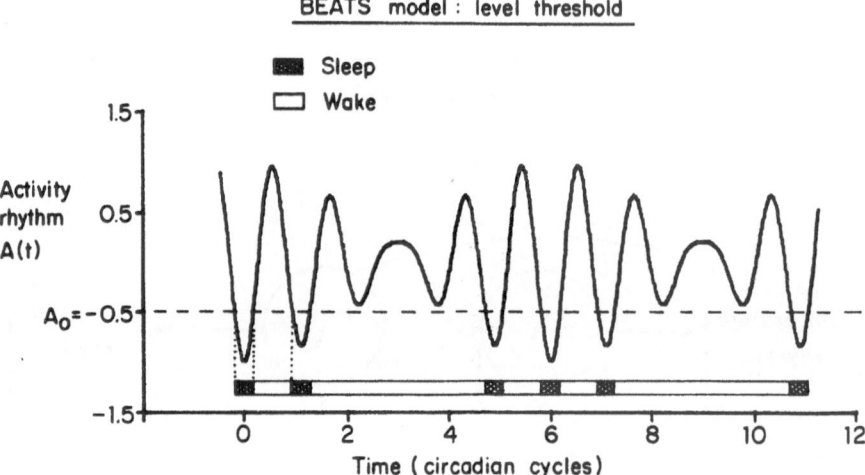

Figure 6-2. Level threshold for BEATS model, following Wever (1979, p. 229). Sleep occurs when activity A falls below a threshold A_0. This threshold criterion sometimes generates unrealistically long wake episodes (e.g. the episode beginning just before circadian cycle #2), due to a reduction in the amplitude of A. This periodic reduction is called a "beat," and occurs here every 5 cycles.

Parameters: $\tau_z = 25$h; $\tau_y = 30$h; (hence $\omega = 5/6$); $a = 0.6$, $b = 1$, $A_0 = -0.5$.

there is a periodic failure of the A rhythm to attain enough amplitude to cross the threshold (Figure 6-2).

Two Level Thresholds

The threshold for sleep onset need not be the same as that for wake-up. An alternative to Wever's (1979) formulation postulates two thresholds, H and L (for high and low). Wake occurs when A crosses H from below, and sleep begins when A crosses L from above. In qualitative terms, this model shares many of the properties of the Daan model; the connection will be made explicit in Section 6.5.

Angular Threshold

Another way to convert the continuous A variable into a binary activity-rest variable involves $\dot{A}$, the time-derivative of A, as well as A itself. This criterion is best understood pictorially (Figure 6-3).

Consider the case when A is free of circadian X modulation, so that $a = 1$ and

$$A = -\cos(\omega t + \gamma) \tag{6.5}$$

$$\dot{A} = \omega \sin(\omega t + \gamma) . \tag{6.6}$$

Then $(A, \dot{A}/\omega)$ transverses a circle clockwise in the $(A, \dot{A}/\omega)$ phase plane. Since people usually sleep about a third of the time, we define sleep as occurring in the $120°$ wedge shown in Figure 6-3.

The wedge is given by

$$\{(A, \dot{A}): A_1, A_2 < 0\} \tag{6.7}$$

where

$$A_1 = -\dot{A}/\omega \tag{6.8}$$

$$A_2 = +\sqrt{3}\, A - \dot{A}/\omega . \tag{6.9}$$

Sleep begins when A_1 crosses down through zero and ends when A_2 crosses up through 0. With the choice of sleep wedge given by (6.8), (6.9) sleep begins near circadian phase 0 during internal synchrony, consistent with observations.

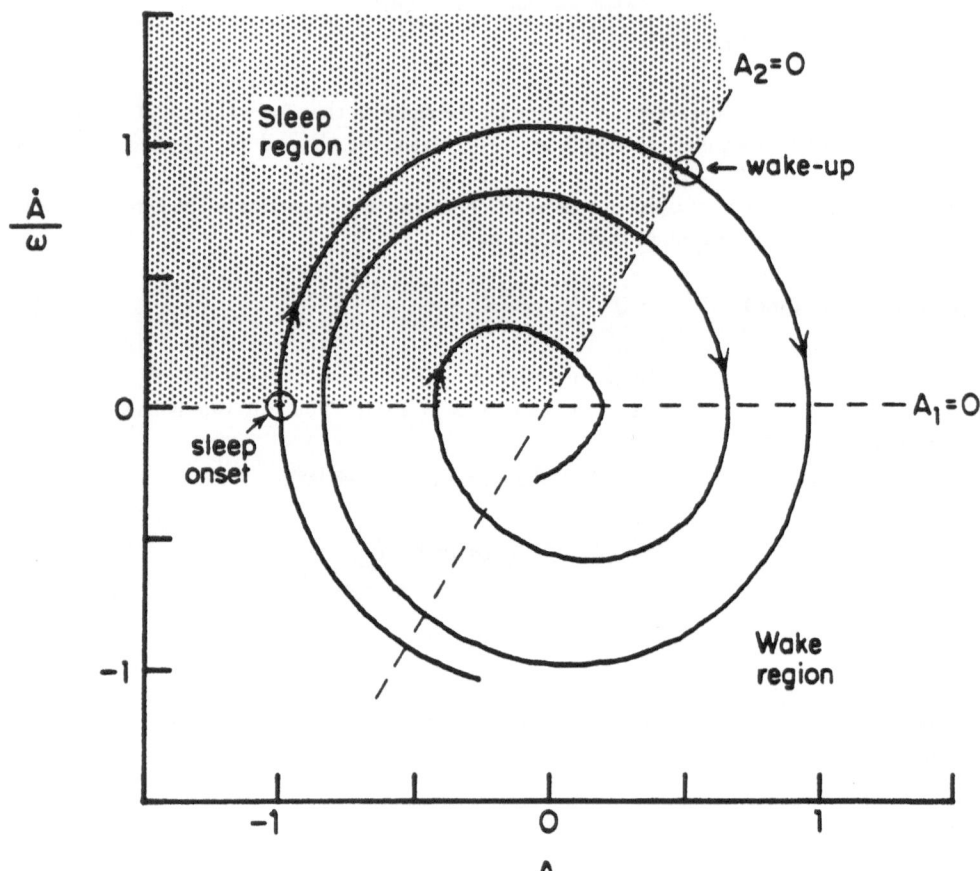

Figure 6-3. Angular threshold for BEATS model. Simulation parameters are those of Figure 6-2, but now sleep occurs in the sector of the $(A, \dot{A}/\omega)$ plane, defined by $A_1 < 0$ and $A_2 < 0$, where A_1 and A_2 are given in equations (6.8), (6.9). Note the low amplitude of A at which the simulation was stopped, corresponding to the occurrence of a beat on circadian cycle #3 (cf. Figure 6-2).

There is an important difference between this angular threshold and the level thresholds, as soon as circadian modulation of A is present: When the X and Y components of A nearly cancel, leading to a small A amplitude, the level threshold will not be crossed and long cycles will result (Figure 6-2); whereas the angular threshold is a *phase* criterion and will produce reasonable results over a wider range of A amplitude. On the other hand, one hallmark deficiency of the angular threshold is its tendency to generate peculiar *short* sleeps, due to low amplitude A rhythms nipping the corner of the wedge (Figure 6-3). For examples of these short sleeps, see Figure 7-1.

6.2.4 Phase Plane Analysis

Many of the properties of the BEATS model can be understood geometrically. Consider the sleep-wake state $P = (A, \dot{A})$ when a circadian component X is present:

$$A = aY + (1-a)X = -a\,\cos(\omega t + \gamma) - (1-a)\cos t \tag{6.10}$$

$$\dot{A} = \omega a\,\sin(\omega t + \gamma) + (1-a)\sin t \ . \tag{6.11}$$

Equations (6.10), (6.11) describe a compound motion: P moves along a "horizontal" ellipse at frequency ω while the center Q of the ellipse follows a circular orbit of frequency 1 (Figure 6-4). The ellipse has major axis of length a, and minor axis of length ωa; thus ω governs its eccentricity. The phase angle γ plays no important geometric role, but merely fixes the initial location of P on the ellipse. The radius of the circle is

$$R = 1 - a \ . \tag{6.12}$$

For conceptual simplicity, the center Q of the ellipse will be taken to reflect the state of the temperature cycle. This is reasonable if the temperature rhythm is almost exclusively controlled by its circadian component, i.e. $b = 1$ in (6.4).

Thus the model has become easy to analyze: The sleep-wake behavior of BEATS is determined by the geometry of Figure 6-4 in conjunction with the choice of thresholds. The phase of the temperature cycle is visible as the center of the ellipse.

The parameter a governs the occurrence of internal desynchronization. That should not be surprising: In the time-series formulation (6.3, 6.4), a measured the proportion of Y in A; when a is large, desynchronization is more likely. Translating into the geometric analysis, a determines the relative sizes of the ellipse and the circle (Figure 6-4). Therefore a determines the access of the state point P to the sleep region of the $(A, \dot{A})$ plane. When a is large, the ellipse intersects the sleep region no matter where the ellipse is centered. This means that for any phase Q of the temperature cycle, there is some point on the ellipse in the sleep region. Sleep is most likely when Q itself lies in the sleep region — this corresponds to the variation of BEDCHECK with circadian phase (Section 4.4.2).

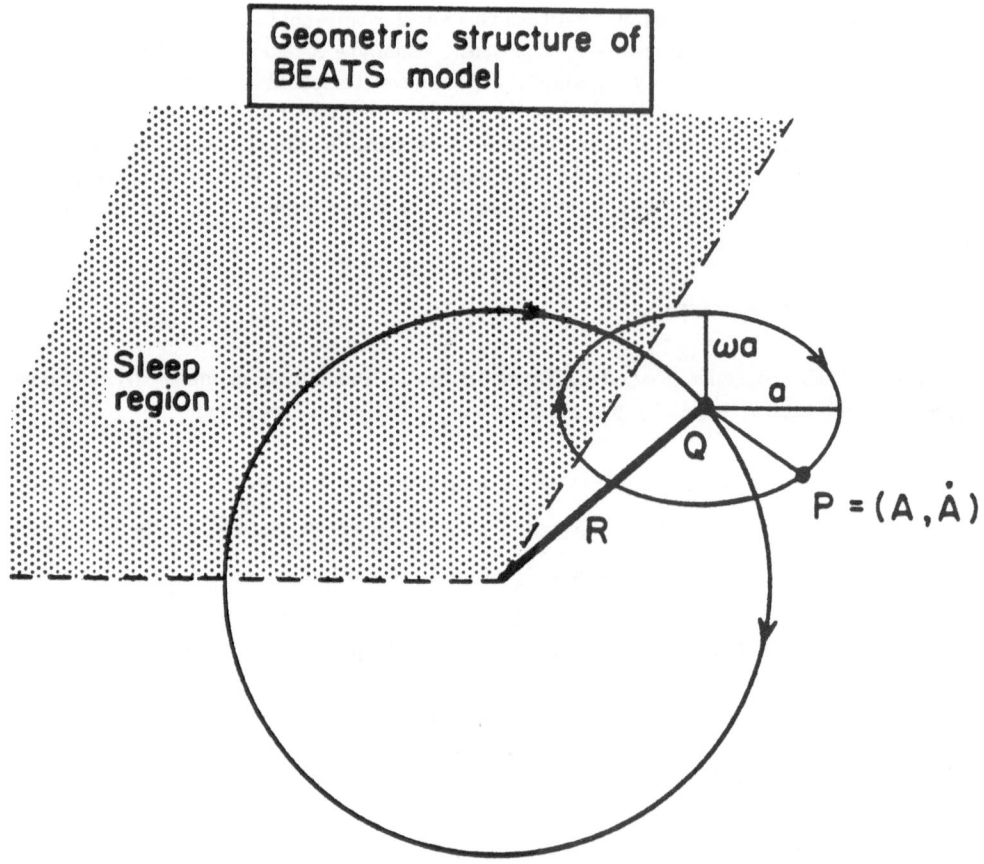

$$Q(t) = (-R\cos t, R\sin t) = \text{circadian component of activity rhythm}$$

$$P(t) = Q(t) + (-a\cos[\omega t + \gamma], \omega a \sin[\omega t + \gamma])$$

$$R = 1 - a = \text{strength of circadian component X of activity rhythm A}$$

Figure 6-4. Geometric structure of the BEATS model (angular threshold version). The state of the system is defined by the point P. P executes a compound motion: it whirls along an ellipse at frequency ω (the frequency of Y), while the center Q of the ellipse traces a circular orbit at frequency 1 (the frequency of the circadian pacemaker X). Sleep occurs when P is in the stippled region. As in Equation (6.10), a and $1-a$ measure the fraction of A due to Y and X, respectively. For example, when $a = 1$, the ellipse grows, the circle shrinks to a point, and sleep occurs at the frequency of Y, with no circadian modulation.

Conversely if a is small, then from many circadian phases Q the ellipse cannot reach the sleep region and so sleep is impossible at those phases. As a decreases, the sleep pattern appears increasingly synchronized. The transition between synchrony and desynchrony is not sharp, but one critical stage for the *level threshold* model occurs when the ellipse can just reach the threshold A_0, even when Q is at its rightmost phase. Let a^* be this critical value. Then

$$a^* = R - A_0 \tag{6.13}$$

$$= 1 - a^* - A_0$$

so

$$a^* = (1 - A_0)/2 \tag{6.14}$$

6.3 PHASE Model

6.3.1 Introduction

We now consider one of the simplest differential equation models of the human circadian system. Like the noninteractive model of the last section, the present model postulates two pacemakers, one manifested by the temperature rhythm and the other by the sleep-wake cycle. The new feature is that the pacemakers are assumed to interact *dynamically*, not merely through a summation of outputs. In other words, the oscillators are coupled. Specifically, we will assume that each oscillator accelerates or slows the other, depending only on their mutual phase relation. Unlike the BEATS model, the present model ignores amplitude and considers only phase. For this reason it will be called the PHASE model.

The PHASE model is studied here for its conceptual simplicity. It introduces the ideas surrounding mutual coupling of oscillators, and it has a mathematically convenient form that allows us to obtain some explicit analytical results. The PHASE model embodies and illuminates the essentials of other coupled oscillator models, e.g. the Van der Pol model of Kronauer *et al.* (1982).

Although no previous authors have applied the model which follows to the human circadian system, the spirit of the model is far from original. Winfree (1980) includes two chapters reviewing and analyzing oscillator models based on phase variables alone. His term for a phase-only oscillator is "simple clock." Ermentrout and Rinzel (1984) discussed loss of entrainment in a simple clock driven by a zeitgeber. Using averaging techniques they derived phase models from more complicated limit cycle dynamics, assuming a weak zeitgeber and a strongly attracting limit cycle. Thus the phase model is a limiting case of general and plausible dynamical schemes. Models of chains of coupled simple clocks have appeared recently, in the context of intestinal frequency plateaus (Ermentrout and Kopell, 1984) and central pattern generators for the swimming of fish (Cohen *et al*, 1982; Kopell, 1986). The work closest to that described below is Hoppensteadt and Keener (1982) or Daan and Berde (1978). The first pair of authors briefly considered a simple clock model of split activity rhythms in rodents, while the second pair studied the same biological problem in more depth, but used difference equations rather than differential equations.

6.3.2 Model Structure

Let θ_1, θ_2 be phases of the two oscillators. Phases are regarded as points on the circle of unit circumference, or equivalently as real numbers, modulo 1. The dynamical equations of the PHASE model are

$$\dot{\theta}_1 = \omega_1 - c_1 \cos 2\pi(\theta_2 - \theta_1)$$

$$\dot{\theta}_2 = \omega_2 + c_2 \cos 2\pi(\theta_1 - \theta_2) \tag{6.15}$$

where ω_1, ω_2 are intrinsic frequencies ($= 1/\tau$, $\tau =$ period)

and c_1, c_2 are coupling strengths.

The overdot signifies time differentiation. All the parameters are taken to be nonnegative. The chosen form of the coupling is such that the first oscillator slows down and the second speeds up when they are in phase. This property is suggested by the observed modulations of sleep-wake cycle lengths ("internal relative coordination," Czeisler, 1978) as the activity and temperature rhythms cross through each other during internal desynchronization.

Returning to equation (6.15), we adopt the conventions that oscillator #1 dominates the temperature rhythm and #2 the sleep-wake cycle. This convention follows Wever's (1975, 1979) Type I/Type II distinction. Thus typically $\omega_1 > \omega_2$. Sleep is defined to occupy some fraction F of the θ_2 circle:

$$\theta_2 = 0 \text{ at sleep onset}$$

$$\theta_2 = F \text{ at wake-up} . \tag{6.16}$$

Here $0 \leq F \leq 1$, and typically $F \sim 1/3$, since people sleep about a third of the time. Since sleep onset during internal synchrony occurs near low temperature, we take $\theta_1 = 0$ as circadian phase 0, the minimum of the endogenous temperature cycle (Figure 6-5).

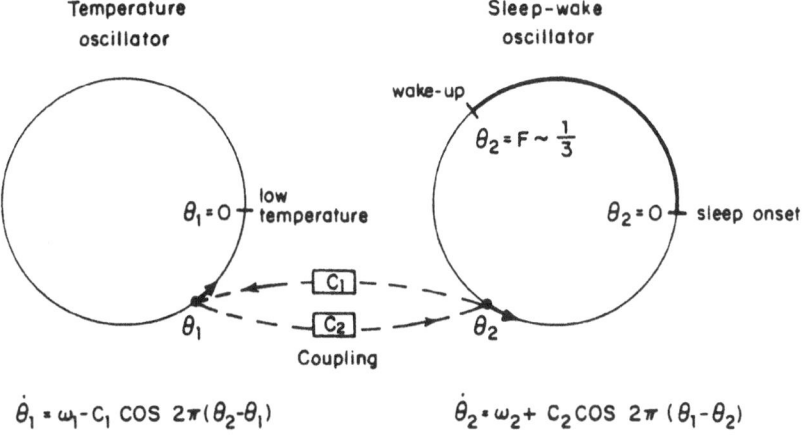

Figure 6-5. Structure of the PHASE model. Sleep-wake and temperature cycles are controlled by different phase-only oscillators, but these oscillators are coupled. Low temperature occurs when $\theta_1 = 0$, and sleep occurs when $\theta_2 \in [0,F]$, where F is a parameter controlling the sleep fraction. Note that all phases are regarded as real numbers (mod 1).

6.3.3 Synchrony

To study the synchronization and desynchronization of the constituent oscillators, consider the phase difference

$$\psi = \theta_1 - \theta_2 \quad . \tag{6.17}$$

Subtracting the equations in (6.15) we see

$$\dot{\psi} = \Omega - c \cos 2\pi\psi \tag{6.18}$$

where

$$\Omega = \omega_1 - \omega_2 \tag{6.19a}$$

$$c = c_1 + c_2 > 0 \quad . \tag{6.19b}$$

Here Ω is the difference of the intrinsic frequencies of the two oscillators and c is the total coupling in the system.

As is reasonable, synchrony is enforced when the coupling c is sufficiently large to offset the frequency difference. Synchrony requires $c > |\Omega|$, so that $\dot{\psi} = 0$ has a solution. Otherwise the phase-difference ψ continues to grow as one oscillator periodically overtakes the other. This desynchronized case will be considered in Section 6.3.4. For now consider the synchronized case, i.e.

$$\text{assume } k = \left| \frac{c}{\Omega} \right| > 1 \quad . \tag{6.20}$$

Then the internally synchronized phase relation ψ^* is obtained by solving (6.18) for $\dot{\psi} = 0$:

$$\psi^* = \pm \frac{1}{2\pi} \cos^{-1} \left(\frac{\Omega}{c} \right) \quad . \tag{6.21}$$

These are two solutions implicit in (6.21); the stable one is that for which $d\dot{\psi}/d\psi < 0$. Here the range of $\cos^{-1}$ is taken as $[0, \pi]$, so

$$\psi^* = (-1/2\pi)\cos^{-1} (\Omega/c)$$

is the stable solution.

Using (6.21) we can also find the "compromise" frequency ω^* adopted by the synchronized system. During internal synchrony, (6.15) becomes

$$\dot{\theta}_1 = \omega_1 - c_1 \left[\frac{\Omega}{c} \right]$$

$$\dot{\theta}_2 = \omega_2 + c_2 \left[\frac{\Omega}{c} \right] .$$

Since $\dot{\theta}_1 = \dot{\theta}_2 = \omega^*$ during synchrony, either of these two expressions simplifies to

$$\omega^* = \frac{c_1 \omega_2 + c_2 \omega_1}{c_1 + c_2} \qquad \text{(synchronized frequency)} . \qquad (6.22)$$

This frequency differs from the intrinsic frequencies ω_1 and ω_2 by amounts $\Delta\omega_1$ and $\Delta\omega_2$:

$$\Delta\omega_1 = \omega^* - \omega_1$$

$$= c_1(\omega_2 - \omega_1)/(c_1 + c_2)$$

$$= -c_1 \Omega/(c_1 + c_2) \qquad (6.23)$$

and

$$\Delta\omega_2 = \omega^* - \omega_2$$
$$= +c_2 \Omega/(c_1 + c_2) . \qquad (6.24)$$

Note that during synchrony the oscillators' frequencies are shifted from their intrinsic values in proportion to the coupling strengths:

$$\left| \frac{\Delta\omega_1}{\Delta\omega_2} \right| = \left| \frac{c_1}{c_2} \right| \qquad (6.25)$$

(Note that results (6.22–6.25) work for more general functions $g(\psi)$, not only $\cos 2\pi\psi$.)

Estimates of the absolute magnitudes of c_1 and c_2 for human subjects are obtained in Section 6.3.5 A.

One important final comment: The PHASE model is incapable of phase-trapping, since ψ cannot oscillate — as Equation (6.18) shows, ψ either monotonically approaches a stable equilibrium (synchrony) or it increases steadily (desynchrony). The inability to phase-trap hinges on the absence of an amplitude variable in the model.

6.3.4 Desynchrony

Equation (6.18) corresponds to desynchrony when $k < 1$, i.e. when $c < |\Omega|$. The phase difference ψ between the oscillators always increases, sometimes slowly and sometimes rapidly, exhibiting what circadian biologists call "internal relative coordination" (Czeisler, 1978; Wever, 1979). The oscillators periodically move through a full cycle of mutual phase relations, with a "beat" frequency β, obtained as follows. From (6.18), the time required for ψ to change from 0 to 1 is $1/\beta$, given by

$$1/\beta = \int_0^{1/\beta} dt = \int_0^1 \frac{d\psi}{\Omega - c \, \cos 2\pi\psi} \tag{6.26}$$

$$= (\Omega^2 - c^2)^{-1/2}$$

(For a derivation of the beat frequency, see Section 6.3.5 B.)

Hence the beat frequency β satisfies

$$\beta = \sqrt{\Omega^2 - c^2} \tag{6.27}$$

$$= \Omega \left[1 - \frac{c^2}{\Omega^2} \right]^{1/2} .$$

Two special cases:

(i) For $c = 0$, the beat frequency reduces to $\beta = \Omega = \omega_1 - \omega_2$, the noninteractive beat frequency as in the BEATS model of Section 6.2.

(ii) As $c \rightarrow \Omega$, $\beta \rightarrow 0$ according to a square root dependence (6.27). Thus the tendency to synchronize grows rapidly as c approaches the critical coupling.

Besides the beat frequency β, another important parameter during desynchrony is the sleep-wake cycle period τ_{SW}. The time τ_{SW} required for θ_2 to complete one cycle is bounded by

$$\frac{1}{\omega_2 + c_2} \leq \tau_{SW} \leq \frac{1}{\omega_2 - c_2} \tag{6.28}$$

(obtained from (6.15), with $\cos 2\pi\psi = \pm 1$).

Equation (6.28) provides crude bounds on τ_{SW}. A more satisfying approach would be to solve (6.15) exactly.

An analytically convenient special case of the model is that in which $c_1 = 0$, i.e. there is no feedback onto the circadian pacemaker. As discussed in Section 4.9.1 this is a reasonable first approximation.

Let the arbitrary zero of time be chosen such that $\theta_1(0) = 0$. Then scaling time such that

$$\omega_1 = 1 \tag{6.29}$$

we obtain

$$\theta_1(t) = t \ . \tag{6.30}$$

As shown in Section 6.3.5 B, equation (6.18) may be solved exactly to yield a complicated (but monotonic and hence invertible) function $\psi(t)$. Rather than writing this function explicitly here, it will be referred to simply as $\psi(t)$.

Having solved for $\theta_1(t)$ and $\psi(t)$, we obtain $\theta_2(t)$:

$$\theta_2(t) = \theta_1(t) - \psi(t)$$

$$= t - \psi(t) \ . \tag{6.31}$$

Model Prediction of $\phi_s{:}\rho$

It would be pleasant if the model's predictions of various empirical relations could be extracted *explicitly* from the model equations. Unfortunately, only *implicit* solutions are possible. For example, consider the model's prediction of $\phi_s{:}\rho$, a pattern discussed in Section 4.1.1. (Recall that ρ is the length of sleep; hence from (6.16), ρ is the time required for θ_2 to move from 0 to F. The phase of sleep onset ϕ_s is given by θ_1, when $\theta_2 = 0$.) To calculate the $\phi_s{:}\rho$ relationship it is most convenient to choose a new origin of time, with $t = 0$ at sleep onset, i.e.

$$\theta_2(0) = 0 \tag{6.32a}$$

$$\theta_1(0) = \phi_s \tag{6.32b}$$

$$\psi(0) = \theta_1(0) - \theta_2(0) = \phi_s \tag{6.32c}$$

Now to find the time at which wake-up occurs, we seek

$$\theta_2(\rho) = F \tag{6.33a}$$

$$\theta_1(\rho) = \phi_s + \rho \tag{6.33b}$$

$$\psi(\rho) = \phi_s + \rho - F . \tag{6.33c}$$

Together (6.32c) and (6.33c) constitute an implicit set of equations for ρ, as a function of ϕ_s and F. Because of the trigonometric form of ψ (see equations (B.14), (B.15) of Section 6.3.5 B), the solution for ρ requires graphical or numerical techniques.

One such graphical method is indicated in Figure 6-6. Equation (6.15) has been numerically integrated to yield the curves $\theta_2(t)$ and $\psi(t)$. Initial conditions were $\theta_1(0) = \theta_2(0) = 0$, and the integration continued until all mutual phase relations ψ between 0 and 1 had been attained. Thus all possible circadian phases of sleep onset are attained, since $\phi_s = \psi$ when $\theta_2 = 0$. To find $\rho(\phi_s)$, we follow a multi-step procedure:

(i) choose ϕ_s, the phase of the sleep onset.

(ii) find t_s such that $\psi(t_s) = \phi_s$. This is always possible since ψ is invertible.

(iii) Regarding t_s as the time of sleep onset, find (the first) t_w such that $\theta_2(t_w) = \theta_2(t_s) + F$.

(iv) Thus t_w represents the time of wake-up and so $\rho = t_w - t_s$. As Figure 6-6b reveals, long sleeps arise when the phase of mid-sleep falls near the inflection point of $\theta_2(t)$. Thus the longest sleeps are predicted to begin in the first half of the circadian cycle (Figure 6-6c), as observed in real data (Section 4.1.1).

Steps (i)–(iv) can be summarized in terms of ψ^{-1} and θ_2^{-1}, the inverse functions to $\psi(t)$ and $\theta_2(t)$, respectively. (We have not yet shown that θ_2 is invertible — see Section 6.3.5 B for the conditions under which it is.) For notational simplicity, let

$$g = \psi^{-1} \quad \text{and} \quad h = \theta_2^{-1} . \tag{6.34}$$

From step (ii),

$$g(\phi_s) = t_s .$$

From step (iii),

$$t_w = h(\theta_2(t_s) + F) = h(\theta_2(g(\phi_s)) + F) . \tag{6.35}$$

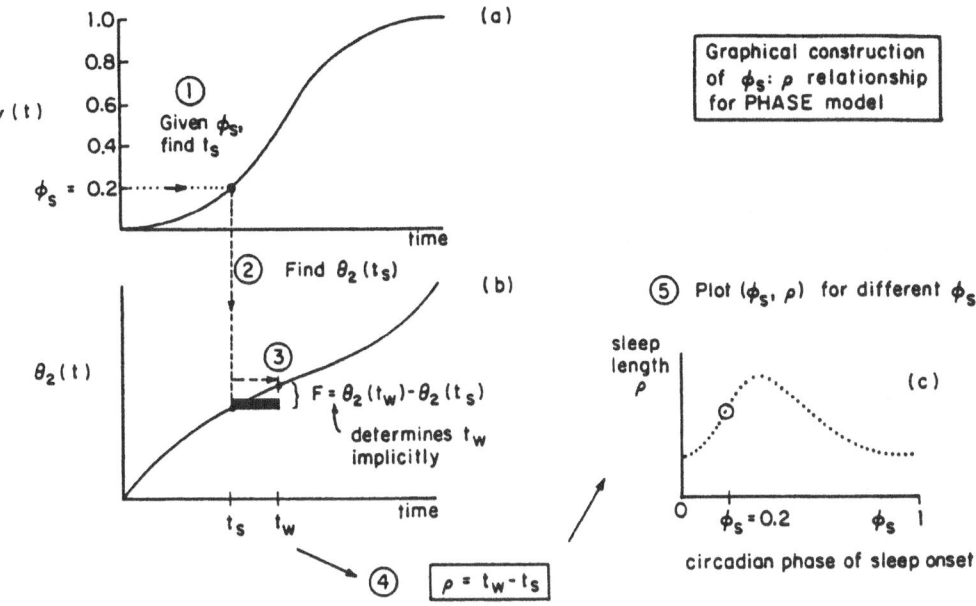

Figure 6-6. Graphical construction of $\phi_s{:}\rho$ (circadian phase of sleep onset: sleep length) in PHASE model. The method is illustrated for $\phi_s = 0.2 = 5$ circadian hours. (a) The time t_s corresponding to $\phi_s = 0.2$ is located on the $\psi(t)$ curve. (b) The phases $\theta_2(t_s)$ and $\theta_2(t_s) + F$ are obtained; they represent the beginning and end of sleep. Wake-up occurs at $t = t_w$; hence sleep length $\rho = t_w - t_s$. (c) The point (ϕ_s, ρ) is plotted, for a sequence of different ϕ_s values.

Thus

$$\rho(\phi_s) = h\left(\theta_2(g(\phi_s)) + F\right) - g(\phi_s) \ . \tag{6.36}$$

Equation (6.36) is the first instance of an exact expression for the $\phi_s{:}\rho$ relation derived from a mathematical model of the sleep-wake cycle.

Model Prediction of $\alpha{:}\rho$

The graphical methods discussed above can also be used to calculate the $\alpha{:}\rho$ relationship implied by the PHASE model. (Recall that α and ρ are the lengths of wake and sleep, respectively.) Fix a point on the $\theta_2(t)$ curve, and then find the times corresponding to $\theta_2(t_s) + F$, and $\theta_2(t_s) + F - 1$. Here t_s is the time of sleep onset, and the two other times just constructed represent the next and the previous wake-up times (Figure 6-7). The cycles indicated in Figure 6-7 fall into roughly 4 classes, parameterized by ϕ_s as in Figure 4-3: (1) On the steep part of $\theta_2(t)$, both α and ρ vary very little over a wide range of ϕ_s. (2) Then ρ starts to lengthen, as does α, but ρ lengthens faster since it approaches the plateau at the inflection point first. Hence both cycle length and sleep fraction increase. (3) After mid-sleep has crossed the plateau of $\theta_2(t)$, ρ must decrease from its maximum while α continues to increase. In this section $\alpha + \rho$ is almost constant. (4) Wake length α achieves its maximum while ρ returns near its minimum value.

The resulting $\alpha{:}\rho$ prediction (Figure 6-7, inset) is triangular, in disagreement with the observations (Section 4.2). The detailed predictions of the model are explored by computer simulations in Chapter 7.

6.3.5 APPENDIX

A. Parameter Estimates for Human Subjects

The earlier equations (6.21)-(6.25) may be used to estimate the coupling strengths c_1, c_2 for typical human subjects. Since the period of the sleep-wake cycle lengthens much more than that of the temperature cycle shortens, we expect

$$c_1 \ll c_2 \ . \tag{A.1}$$

Since $\Omega = c$ at the onset of desynchrony, and $c = c_1 + c_2 \sim c_2$, the frequency difference Ω provides an estimate of c_2:

$$c_2 \sim \text{frequency difference } \Omega \text{ observed at onset of desynchrony.} \tag{A.2}$$

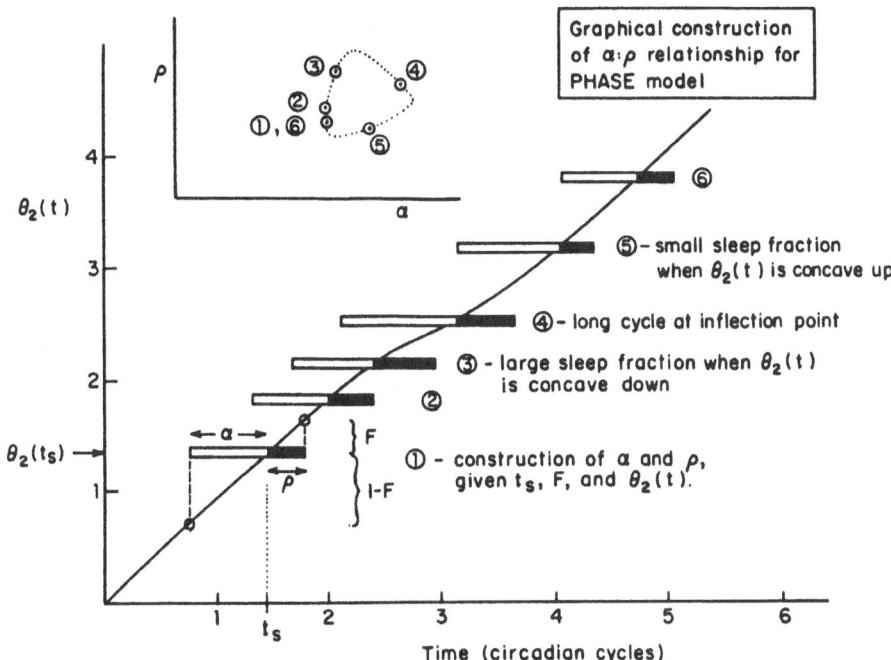

Figure 6-7. Graphical construction of $\alpha{:}\rho$ relationship for PHASE model. The curve $\theta_2(t)$ and sleep fraction parameter F are assumed given. For any time t_s of sleep onset, the times corresponding to $\theta_2 = \theta_2(t_s) + F - 1$, and $\theta_2 = \theta_2(t_s) + F$ are located; these mark the beginning of the preceding wake and the end of the current sleep, and hence define α and ρ. Six different choices of t_s, and the resulting $\alpha{:}\rho$ relationship (inset, upper left) are shown.

Choosing units where $\omega_1 = 1$, a typical value for Ω would be

$$\Omega \sim 1/6 \sim 0.16 \quad (\sim 6 \text{ day beat period}) \ . \tag{A.3}$$

Hence,

$$c_2 \sim 0.16 \ . \tag{A.4}$$

From (6.24), (A.1), and (A.3),

$$\Delta\omega_2 \sim 0.16 \ . \tag{A.5}$$

To obtain c_1, we recall Wever's (1979) result that after desynchrony, the temperature cycle shortens by ~ 0.7 h. For a synchronized period of 25.5 h, this corresponds to

$$\omega^* = 24.8/25.5 = 0.97 \ . \tag{A.6}$$

Since

$$\Delta\omega_1 = \omega^* - \omega_1$$

$$\sim 0.97 - 1.0$$

$$\sim -0.03 \tag{A.7}$$

we find from (11) that

$$c_1 = |c_2 \Delta\omega_1/\Delta\omega_2|$$

$$\sim 0.03 \quad . \tag{A.8}$$

Hence the couplings are in a ratio of

$$|c_1/c_2| \sim |0.03/0.16| \sim 1/5 \ . \tag{A.9}$$

B. Exact Solution for θ_1 and θ_2

We consider the system

$$\dot{\theta}_1 = 1 \tag{B.1}$$

$$\dot{\theta}_2 = w + c \, \cos \, 2\pi(\theta_1 - \theta_2) \ .$$

This system subsumes equation (6.15) of Section 6.3.2, for the case $c_1 = 0$. Time is scaled so that $w_1 = 1$; then w_2 becomes w and c_2 becomes c, in these new units.

Let

$$\psi = \theta_1 - \theta_2 \ . \tag{B.2}$$

Then

$$\dot{\psi} = 1 - w - c \, \cos \, 2\pi\psi \tag{B.3}$$

$$= \Omega - c \, \cos \, 2\pi\psi \tag{B.4}$$

where

$$\Omega = 1 - w \ . \tag{B.5}$$

Rescale time again: Set

$$T = \Omega t \tag{B.6}$$

and let

$$\psi' = d\psi/dT \ . \tag{B.7}$$

Then

$$\psi' = 1 - k \, \cos \, 2\pi\psi \tag{B.8}$$

where

$$k = c/\Omega .$$

(B.9)

Here k represents a dimensionless coupling constant; desynchrony occurs when

$$k < 1 .$$

(B.10)

Equation (B.8) can be solved by separation of variables, followed by integration. Using the substitution

$$x = \tan \pi\psi$$

(B.11)

we obtain

$$T + \text{constant} = \int \frac{d\psi}{1 - k \cos 2\pi\psi}$$

$$= \left(\frac{1}{\pi(1+k)b} \right) \arctan(x/b)$$

(B.12)

where

$$b^2 = (1-k)/(1+k) .$$

(B.13)

Equation (B.12) may be solved for x and then for ψ to yield

$$\psi(t) = \frac{1}{\pi} \arctan u(t)$$

(B.14)

where:

$$u(t) = b \tan(\pi\beta t + C_0)$$

(B.15)

$\beta = \Omega(1-k^2)^{1/2}$ is the beat frequency

(B.16)

$$C_0 = \arctan \left| \frac{1}{b} \tan \pi\psi_0 \right|$$

(B.17)

$\psi_0 = \psi(t{=}0)$ is the initial condition $\hspace{4cm}$ (B.18)

$b^2 = (1{-}k)/(1{+}k)$ $\hspace{6cm}$ (B.19)

$k = c/(1{-}\omega)$ is the dimensionless coupling . $\hspace{3cm}$ (B.20)

The equations (B.14)–(B.20) solve the equation given by (B.3) for the desynchronized case assumed in (B.10). Then θ_1 and θ_2 are easily solved for, as shown in equations (6.30), (6.31) of Section 6.3.4.

Monotonicity of $\theta_2(t)$

Around the discussion of Figure 6-6, it was stated that $\theta_2(t)$ is a monotonic function of t, for certain reasonable choices of parameters. All that is required in fact, is $c < |\Omega|$ (the condition characterizing desynchrony) and $\omega_2 > 1/2$ (activity rhythm period is less than bicircadian).

Proof:

$$\omega_2 > \frac{1}{2} \;\longrightarrow\; \omega_2 > 1 - \omega_2$$

$$\longrightarrow\; \omega_2 > \Omega \quad \text{(from (6.29) and (6.19a))}$$

$$\longrightarrow\; \omega_2 + \Omega \cos 2\pi\psi > 0 \quad \text{for all } \psi$$

$$\longrightarrow\; \omega_2 + c_2 \cos 2\pi\psi > 0, \quad \text{since } c_2 \leq c < |\Omega|$$

$$\longrightarrow\; \dot{\theta}_2 > 0 \quad \text{(from (6.15))}$$

$$\longrightarrow\; \theta_2(t) \quad \text{is monotone in } t, \text{ as required .}$$

As a corollary, the $\rho(\phi_s)$ curve is continuous: the graphical argument of Figure 6-6b shows that discontinuities in ρ arise only at points where $\dot{\theta}_2(t_w) = 0$. Hence in the PHASE model, desynchrony with a discontinuous $\phi_s{:}\rho$ relation is impossible until τ_2 exceeds bicircadian lengths.

6.4 XY Model of Kronauer *et al.*

This section analyzes the XY model of free-run by asymptotic methods. The analysis involves an averaging technique (Minorsky 1962; Stoker, 1950) called the stroboscopic method (Minorsky, 1962, Chapter 16). The upshot is that the PHASE model (Section 6.3) and the BEATS model (Section 6.2) may be regarded as different limiting cases of the more complex XY model.

6.4.1 Simplifying the Equations

The equations for the XY model (Kronauer *et al.*, 1982, 1983; Kronauer, 1984) are conventionally written in the form

$$k^2\ddot{x} + k\mu_x(x^2-1)\dot{x} + (24/\hat{\tau}_x)^2 x + F_{yx}k\dot{y} = 0 \tag{6.37}$$

$$k^2\ddot{y} + k\mu_y(y^2-1)\dot{y} + (24/\hat{\tau}_y)^2 y + F_{xy}k\dot{x} = 0 \tag{6.38}$$

where $k = 24/2\pi$ allows time to be expressed in hours. For analysis this choice of units is less convenient than a nondimensional time. Scaling time by

$$\tilde{t} = 24t/k\hat{\tau}_x = (2\pi/\hat{\tau}_x)t \tag{6.39}$$

the equations become

$$\ddot{x} + \epsilon(x^2-1)\dot{x} + x + (F_{yx}/\hat{\omega}_x)\dot{y} = 0 \tag{6.40}$$

$$\ddot{y} + \epsilon(y^2-1)\dot{y} + (1+\epsilon\nu)y + (F_{xy}/\hat{\omega}_x)\dot{x} = 0 \tag{6.41}$$

where the overdot now means $d/d\tilde{t}$;

$$\hat{\omega}_x = 24/\hat{\tau}_x \quad, \tag{6.42}$$

$$\epsilon\nu = (\hat{\tau}_x/\hat{\tau}_y)^2 - 1 \quad, \tag{6.43}$$

and

$$\epsilon = \mu_x/\hat{\omega}_x = \mu_y/\hat{\omega}_x \quad. \tag{6.44}$$

(Here we have used the equality $\mu_x = \mu_y = 0.1$ assumed by Kronauer *et al.* (1982).) Define dimensionless couplings C_{xy}, C_{yx} by

$$\epsilon C_{xy} = F_{xy}/\hat{\omega}_x \tag{6.45}$$

$$\epsilon C_{yx} = F_{yx}/\hat{\omega}_x \tag{6.46}$$

so that the equations simplify to

$$\ddot{x} + x + \epsilon f(x,\dot{x},y,\dot{y}) = 0 \tag{6.47}$$

$$\ddot{y} + y + \epsilon g(x,\dot{x},y,\dot{y}) = 0 \tag{6.48}$$

where

$$f = (x^2-1)\dot{x} + C_{yx}\dot{y} \tag{6.49}$$

$$g = (y^2-1)\dot{y} + \nu y + C_{xy}\dot{x} \quad . \tag{6.50}$$

6.4.2 Stroboscopic Analysis

For small ϵ the equations (6.47, 6.48) may be analyzed by the stroboscopic method (Minorsky, 1962). This method gives asymptotic equations for the slow variations (time scale $= \epsilon t$) of the amplitude and phase of x and y, as follows.

Define new variables r_1, θ_1, r_2, θ_2 according to

$$x = r_1\cos(t+\theta_1) \qquad y = r_2\cos(t+\theta_2)$$

$$\tag{6.51}$$

$$\dot{x} = -r_1\sin(t+\theta_1) \qquad \dot{y} = -r_2\sin(t+\theta_2) \quad .$$

The r and θ variables are functions of time and represent slowly varying amplitudes and phases, respectively. Their time evolution is governed by the stroboscopic equations

$$\dot{r}_1 = \epsilon\langle f \, \sin(t+\theta_1)\rangle \tag{6.52a}$$

$$\dot{r}_2 = \epsilon\langle g \, \sin(t+\theta_2)\rangle \tag{6.52b}$$

$$r_1\dot{\theta}_1 = \epsilon\langle f \, \cos(t+\theta_1)\rangle \tag{6.52c}$$

$$r_2\dot{\theta}_2 = \epsilon\langle g \, \cos(t+\theta_2)\rangle \tag{6.52d}$$

where the averaging operator $\langle \cdot \rangle$ is defined by

$$\langle h(t)\rangle = \frac{1}{2\pi} \int\limits_{t-\pi}^{t+\pi} h(s) \, ds \quad . \tag{6.53}$$

Substituting (6.49, 6.51) into (6.52a), we obtain

$$\dot{r}_1 = \epsilon\langle [r_1^2\cos^2(t+\theta_1)-1]r_1\sin^2(t+\theta_1) - C_{yz}r_2\sin(t+\theta_1)\sin(t+\theta_2)\rangle \quad . \tag{6.54}$$

Using the averaging relations

$$\langle \cos^2\sin^2\rangle = \frac{1}{8}$$

$$\langle \sin^2\rangle = \frac{1}{2}$$

$$\langle \sin(t+\theta_1)\sin(t+\theta_2)\rangle = \frac{1}{2}\langle \cos(\theta_1-\theta_2) - \cos(2t+\theta_1+\theta_2)\rangle$$

$$= \frac{1}{2}\cos(\theta_1-\theta_2)$$

(6.54) reduces to

$$\frac{\dot{r}_1}{\epsilon} = \frac{r_1}{2} - \frac{r_1^3}{8} - \frac{C_{yz}}{2}\,r_2\cos(\theta_1-\theta_2) \quad .$$

Similar averaging and simplification of (6.52) leads to the full set of slow time equations:

$$r_1' = \frac{r_1}{2} - \frac{r_1^3}{8} - \frac{C_{yz}}{2} r_2 \cos(\theta_1 - \theta_2) \tag{6.55a}$$

$$r_2' = \frac{r_2}{2} - \frac{r_2^3}{8} - \frac{C_{zy}}{2} r_1 \cos(\theta_2 - \theta_1) \tag{6.55b}$$

$$r_1 \theta_1' = \frac{C_{yz}}{2} r_2 \sin(\theta_1 - \theta_2) \tag{6.55c}$$

$$r_2 \theta_2' = - \frac{C_{zy}}{2} r_1 \sin(\theta_1 - \theta_2) + \frac{\nu r_2}{2} \tag{6.55d}$$

where differentiation with respect to "slow-time" ϵt is denoted by the prime symbol $'$.

6.4.3 Weak Coupling and Detuning Imply a PHASE Model

Further simplifications result from assuming that the couplings C_{zy}, C_{yz} and the detuning ν are weak:

$$C_{zy} , \ C_{yz} , \ \nu \ll 1 . \tag{6.56}$$

Then from (6.55) the phases θ_1 and θ_2 vary on super-slow time scales $O(\epsilon C t)$ or $O(\epsilon \nu t)$, while the amplitudes r_1 and r_2 vary on the more rapid scale $O(\epsilon t)$. Assume that the amplitudes have nearly reached equilibrium, so that both x and y are close to their limit cycles:

$$r_1 = 2 + \delta_1 \tag{6.57}$$

$$r_2 = 2 + \delta_2 \tag{6.58}$$

with

$$\delta_1 , \ \delta_2 \ll 1 . \tag{6.59}$$

Substituting (6.57, 6.58) into (6.55) yields

$$\delta_1' = -\delta_1 - C_{yx} \cos(\theta_1 - \theta_2) \tag{6.60a}$$

$$\delta_2' = -\delta_2 - C_{xy} \cos(\theta_1 - \theta_2) \tag{6.60b}$$

$$\theta_1' = \frac{C_{yx}}{2} \sin(\theta_1 - \theta_2) \tag{6.60c}$$

$$\theta_2' = -\frac{C_{xy}}{2} \sin(\theta_1 - \theta_2) + \frac{\nu}{2} \, . \tag{6.60d}$$

In (6.60), quadratic terms of order $O(C\delta)$, $O(\delta^2)$ and $O(\nu\delta)$ have been neglected.

Note that to this order of approximation, the equations (6.60c,d) reduce to a "phase model" (Section 6.3) — θ_1' and θ_2' are independent of amplitude deviations δ_1 and δ_2. Subtracting (6.60d) from (6.60c) yields an equation for the phase difference ψ:

$$\psi = \theta_1 - \theta_2 \tag{6.61}$$

$$\psi' = \frac{1}{2} \left(C_{xy} + C_{yx} \right) \sin \psi + \frac{\nu}{2} \, . \tag{6.62}$$

This equation may be analyzed by the methods of Section 6.3, and parameters relevant to human data may be estimated by the methods of Section 6.3.5 A.

6.4.4 Relation between XY and BEATS Models

A perturbation analysis presented by Stoker (1950, pp. 163-171) addresses the response of a Van der Pol oscillator forced at a frequency ω_1 different from its intrinsic frequency ω_0. The amplitude of the forcing is held fixed while the frequency difference ("detuning") is varied. At small detuning, the oscillator is entrained at frequency ω_1; at large detuning, there is essentially the unforced response at frequency ω_0. The case of interest to us occurs between these two extremes: at intermediate detuning the response is a "combination oscillation" composed of free and forced modes beating together. As in the BEATS model (Section 6.2) these modes are simple harmonic oscillations at frequencies ω_0 and ω_1. Thus these observations connect the forced Van der Pol to the BEATS model.

The further connection between the forced Van der Pol and the XY model arises from the observation that in (6.37, 6.38), $F_{xy} \gg F_{yx}$. That is, x may be regarded as forcing y yet receiving little feedback (Kronauer et al. 1982) so that Stoker's analysis applies, to a first approximation. Thus the XY and BEATS models are related, through their common connection to the forced Van der Pol system.

6.5 Model of Daan *et al.*

6.5.1 Introduction

This section explores the gated pacemaker model proposed by Daan and Beersma (1984) and refined by Daan *et al.* (1984). For an overview of the model structure and published results, see Section 5.6.

The first version of the model (Daan and Beersma, 1984) involved pure sinusoidal thresholds. The authors remarked that the choice of sinusoidal modulation was arbitrary, and that in several respects the model's performance could be improved by skewing the wake-up threshold to rise more steeply and fall more slowly than a sine wave. The threshold's precise shape was derived from the sleep deprivation data of Akerstedt and Gillberg (1981). In the second version of their model, Daan *et al.* (1984) incorporated the skewed threshold. Henceforth both versions of the model will be called DAAN; when it is helpful to distinguish between them, the first will be called SINE and the second SKEW.

The seemingly pedantic distinction between SINE and SKEW turns out to be important in connection to unsuccessful attempts to reproduce the results of Daan *et al.* (1984). There is a substantial oversight in Daan *et al.* (1984), as graciously acknowledged by Professor Serge Daan (personal communication, Sept. 1985).

Comparison of the reported ϕ_s:ρ prediction of SKEW (Figure 11, Daan *et al.*, 1984) with that of SINE (Figure 10, Daan and Beersma, 1984) reveals that the figures are *identical*, even though reportedly made by two different models. Somehow the old results from SINE were used in place of the new results from SKEW. Professor Serge Daan kindly acknowledged this accidental substitution. He also confirmed that my SKEW simulations of the ϕ_s:ρ plot agreed with his and that the new results were inferior to those of the original SINE model.

6.5.2 Altered Threshold Parameters

As mentioned above, the current parameters used in SKEW lead to an incorrect prediction of the ϕ_s:ρ relationship. Daan (personal communication, Sept. 1985) suggested that the problem could be remedied by introducing more variability in the upper threshold H.

However, it seems that the main problem with the original parameters of SKEW (Daan *et al.*, 1984) is that the mean level $\overline{L}$ of the lower threshold is too large ($\overline{L} = 0.16 - 0.17$). With a smaller value of $\overline{L}$, the data from internal desynchrony can be better accommodated.

As a rough way to estimate appropriate values of $\overline{H}$ and $\overline{L}$, we can derive exact solutions for the sleep-wake cycle period and for the sleep fraction, in the case of zero circadian modulation, i.e., *flat* thresholds ($A_H = A_L = 0$).

At time 0, suppose $S = \overline{H}$, i.e. $S_0 = \overline{H}$. How long does it take for S to fall to $\overline{L}$? At the n-th half-hour step

$$S_n = d^n S_0 = d^n \bar{H} \tag{6.63}$$

where $d = 0.888$ is the decay rate of S. (See Section 5.6.) S strikes the lower threshold when $S_n = \bar{L}$, i.e., when

$$\bar{L} = d^n \bar{H} \; .$$

Solving for n we obtain

$$n = \log(\bar{L}/\bar{H})/\log d \; .$$

Since each step is 0.5 h, the predicted sleep length ρ satisfies

$$\rho = 0.5 \, \frac{\log(\bar{L}/\bar{H})}{\log d} \; . \tag{6.64}$$

Using a similar approach to calculate the wake length α we find

$$\alpha = 0.5 \, \frac{\log \left(\dfrac{1-\bar{H}}{1-\bar{L}} \right)}{\log u} \tag{6.65}$$

where $u = 0.973 =$ rise rate of S during wakefulness.

Equations (6.64) and (6.65) allow us to calculate the cycle length τ_{SW} and the sleep fraction F according to

$$\tau_{SW} = \alpha + \rho = \text{wake–sleep cycle length} \tag{6.66}$$

$$F = \rho/(\alpha+\rho) = \text{sleep fraction} \; . \tag{6.67}$$

Figure 6-8 is a contour map on the $\bar{L}{:}\bar{H}$ plane, showing curves of constant sleep fraction, and also curves of constant cycle length. Only parameters relevant to internal desynchrony are shown. As expected, it is mainly the $\bar{H} - \bar{L}$ separation which determines τ_{SW}, and the average level $(\bar{H} + \bar{L})/2$ which determines F. Large separation of thresholds leads to large τ_{SW}, and a large average level leads to decreased sleep fraction (since S falls more rapidly than it rises, and the discrepancy increases with S.)

From Figure 6-8, it is evident that $\bar{L} = 0.16$ (as in Daan et al., 1984) is on the upper border of acceptable values. It tends to produce small sleep fractions. Of course, the results given here will be modified by circadian modulation in the thresholds, but for reasonably

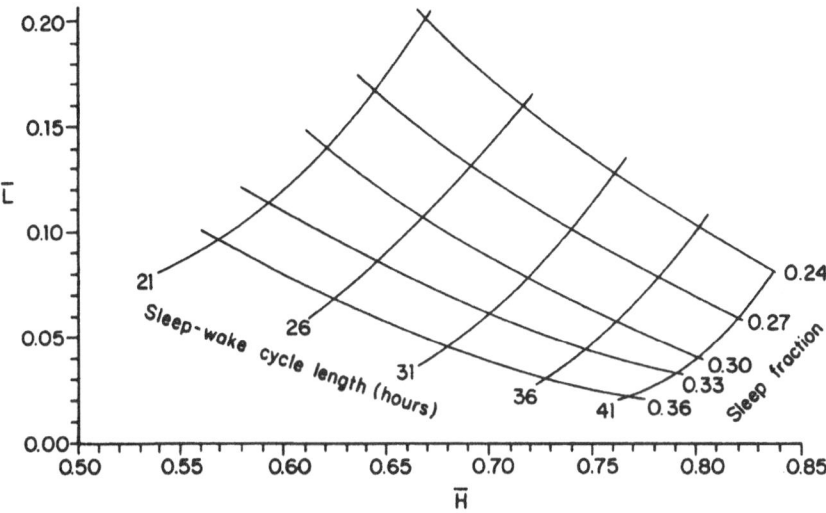

Figure 6-8. Contour map of sleep-wake cycle length τ_{SW} and sleep fraction F for the DAAN model, assuming flat thresholds ($A = 0$, i.e., no circadian modulation). Only the region relevant to internal desynchronization is shown. The τ_{SW} and F contours have slopes ~ 1 and $\sim -1/2$, respectively.

small amplitudes our expectations of τ_{SW} and F are not too far off, as the simulations of Chapter 7 demonstrate.

6.5.3 Phase Plane Analysis

To compare the geometric underpinnings of DAAN to models we have considered previously, it is helpful to construct a phase plane representation of the model. First, the kinetics are

$$\dot{S} = -dS \quad (\text{decay of } S = \text{sleep}) \qquad (6.68)$$

$$\dot{S} = r - rS \quad (\text{rise of } S = \text{wake}) \qquad (6.69)$$

Recall that the decay is faster than the rise, i.e.

$$|d| > |r| \qquad (6.70)$$

Thus in the $(S, \dot{S})$ phase plane (Figure 6-9) the system drifts along the "awake" line, crosses threshold H, jumps down to the "asleep" line, drifts back again, then crosses the wake-up threshold L and returns to its starting state.

The thresholds H and L appear as fixed lines in the phase plane, assuming zero circadian modulation. The more complicated case of nonzero modulation can be visualized in two ways: (i) the vertical lines $(S = H$ and $S = L)$ oscillate about their mean positions given by the fixed vertical lines $S = \bar{H}$ and $S = \bar{L}$. Sometimes the state point $P = (S, \dot{S})$ collides head-on with the onrushing threshold, or it overtakes the slowly retreating threshold — in either case, wake-up occurs when P crosses the moving wake-up threshold, and similarly for bedtime. (ii) Rather than picturing a moving threshold, it may be easier to imagine *fixed* thresholds, with the lines (6.68, 6.69) defined relative to a *moving* origin. The double-rail track of Figure 6-9 is pushed back and forth along the S axis, at the circadian frequency ω. To separate the forward from backward motion, we use the vertical dimension of the phase plane to depict the velocity of the track (Figure 6-9). The track moves left to right along the top of the ellipse. Meanwhile the state point P continues to move around the two-rail track. Wake-up occurs when $S = L$ (and $\dot{S} < 0$); assuming $L = \bar{L} - A \cos \omega t$, the condition for wake-up is

$$S + A \cos \omega t = \bar{L} \qquad (6.71)$$

Equation (6.71) may be visualized in Figure 6-9; the x-coordinate of the system is $S + A \cos \omega t$, due to the combined motion of the system around the track, and of the track itself around the ellipse.

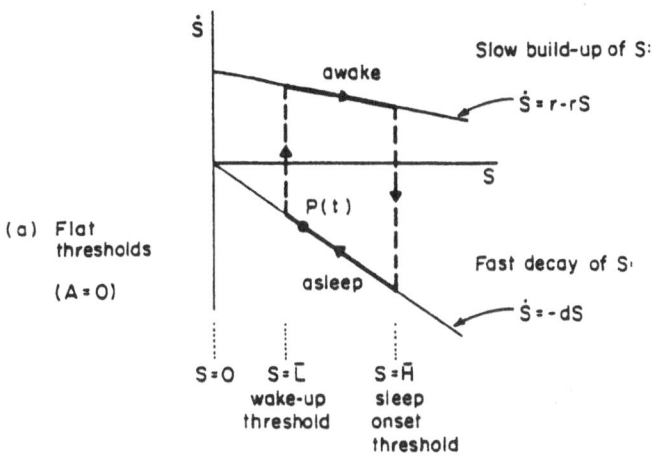

(a) Flat thresholds

(A = 0)

Slow build-up of S:

$\dot{S} = r - rS$

Fast decay of S:

$\dot{S} = -dS$

$S = 0$ $S = L$ $S = H$
wake-up   sleep
threshold   onset
threshold

(b) Effect of circadian modulation of thresholds

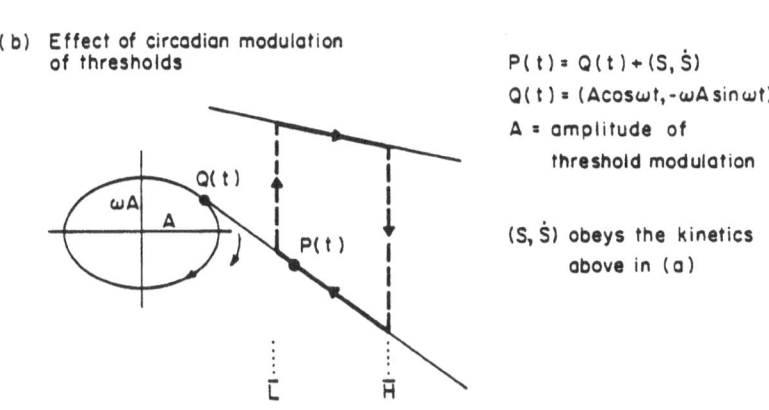

$P(t) = Q(t) + (S, \dot{S})$

$Q(t) = (A\cos\omega t, -\omega A \sin\omega t)$

A = amplitude of threshold modulation

$(S, \dot{S})$ obeys the kinetics above in (a)

Figure 6-9. Phase plane representation of DAAN model.

(a) Without circadian modulation the thresholds H and L reduce to fixed vertical lines $S = H$ and $S = L$ in the $(S,\dot{S})$ phase plane. The state of the S process at time t is represented by the point $P(t)$. It is confined to motion along the two lines indicated ("rails"), except for instantaneous jumps between the rails whenever a threshold is reached.

(b) The phase plane representation of (a) is modified by a sinusoidal circadian modulation of the thresholds. Point P still moves only along the rails, and jumps between them upon crossing one of the fixed thresholds; but the rails are no longer fixed in the plane. Instead they are rigidly transported around a small elliptical track (exaggerated for clarity). Thus P executes a compound motion, due partly to the relaxation kinetics of the S process along the rails, and partly to the circadian orbital motion of the rails themselves. This compound motion recalls the BEATS model; compare Figure 6-4.

6.5.4 Connection to Other Models

Perhaps the previous construction seems contrived. However, it does reveal the essential similarities and differences of DAAN and models we have considered earlier. Compare the phase plane of the BEATS model (Section 6.2.4). In BEATS, the state point moves along an ellipse, whose center follows a circular orbit (Figure 6-4). In DAAN, the state point is confined to a double-rail track, instead of an ellipse (Figure 6-9). Two vertical lines represent thresholds in both models (here, we are using the two level threshold version of BEATS — Section 6.2.3). Upon crossing a threshold, DAAN jumps to the opposite rail, whereas BEATS simply continues around the ellipse with no discontinuities of state.

Another difference between the models involves the velocity of the state point: DAAN has a monotone increasing or decreasing velocity on each rail of its track, whereas BEATS speeds up *and* slows down on each section of its ellipse.

Finally note that through BEATS, we have connected the DAAN and XY models (see Section 6.4.4). All three models involve compound motion: the state point moves along a track which itself executes a circadian orbit in the phase plane. But the shapes of the tracks are different: elliptical (BEATS, XY) or two rails with jumps (DAAN). Moreover, the threshold criteria are either angular (XY, angular version of BEATS) or two flat thresholds (DAAN, two threshold version of BEATS).

Chapter 7

Simulations

Introduction

The previous chapters have set the stage for a confrontation of experiment and theory. Chapter 3 presented many records of internally desynchronized subjects, regarded individually and in all their particulars. Chapter 4 extracted from those records certain generalizations, empirical patterns that underlie the timing of the sleep-wake cycle under free-running conditions. Turning from experiment to theory, Chapter 5 reviewed previous models of the sleep-wake cycle, and Chapter 6 explored the analytical structure of the two leading contenders: the XY model of Kronauer *et al.* (1982, 1983) and the gated pacemaker model of Daan *et al.* (1984). Chapter 6 also introduced two simpler alternative models, BEATS and PHASE, with a dual purpose. First, they were used in Chapter 6 to illuminate the structure of the more sophisticated models. In this chapter, they act as "controls" during tests of the models. That is, the BEATS and PHASE models offer a standard of performance, against which the sophisticated models are measured. The models of Daan *et al.* and Kronauer *et al.* are to be judged successful, not when they reproduce some empirical pattern, but when they reproduce it more faithfully than the control models do.

Overview of Chapter 7

Computer simulation programs were written for each of the four classes of models examined below. Simulations of the models generate a body of synthetic sleep-wake and temperature data, which can be analyzed in the same manner as actual human data. Thus, the models are tested by comparing these synthetic data to the experimental results of Chapters 3 and 4.

Raster plots are presented in Section 7.1 to show each model's version of the transition from synchrony to desynchrony. Section 7.2 presents simulations of napping and split-sleep patterns (Section 4.10), phenomena which none of the models were designed to address. In this way we gauge their relative performances in unfamiliar territory, and not only their *post hoc* consistency. Next, model predictions about internal desynchronization are studied in detail. Section 7.3 compares simulations of a representative desynchrony — the models are checked for their qualitative accuracy, i.e., their capacity to account for the *form* of the relationships of Chapter 4. Section 7.4 pushes the models a bit harder by testing their quantitative accuracy. The approach is to run a number of simulations over a range of parameters, and to pool the resulting synthetic data, analogous to the treatment of the human data in Chapter 4. The results are summarized and discussed in Section 7.5.

7.1 Transition from Synchrony to Desynchrony

Mechanisms for spontaneous internal desynchronization have been proposed by Kronauer *et al.* (1982) and Daan *et al.* (1984). In the "coupled limit cycle oscillator" model of

Kronauer *et al.*, the intrinsic period $\hat{\tau}_y$ of the sleep-wake oscillator is postulated to lengthen during prolonged temporal isolation, until it is outside the range of entrainment of the x oscillator. In the "relaxation oscillator plus modulated threshold" model of Daan *et al.*, the amplitude of the circadian modulation is postulated to decrease spontaneously in free-run. At sufficiently weak modulation, internal synchronization is lost. The qualitative character of synchrony loss in these two models, and in the two simpler models, PHASE and BEATS, is shown in Figure 7-1.

The parameters used in the simulations of Figure 7-1 are given in the legend to Figure 7-1. In all cases, some parameter was assumed to drift throughout the simulation.

The scenario in the XY model (Figure 7-1a) is familiar (Kronauer *et al.*, 1982; Moore-Ede *et al.*, 1982). The x and y rhythms are synchronized for the first 10 cycles, then internal phase drift sets in as $\hat{\tau}_y$ lengthens and y pulls away from x. Around cycle 35 there is phase-trapping (Section 4.7), ending with the characteristic short sleep (cycle 44) that signals a low amplitude of y and the boundary between synchrony and desynchrony.

The model of Daan *et al.* (Figure 7-1b) also shows internal phase drift in this case as the modulation amplitude decreases. Desynchrony occurs around cycle 35, without intermediate phase-trapping.

The PHASE model (Figure 7-1c) also shows internal phase drift, less than the XY model and comparable to the DAAN model. Also like the DAAN model, PHASE shows no phase-trapping before desynchrony.

The BEATS model (Figure 7-1d) is based on a summation of sinusoids and hence never truly synchronizes. That is, the sleep-wake rhythm always contains *two* noninteracting frequency components, corresponding to the X and Y inputs. Therefore, phase-trapping is present from the start, and it builds up as the activity rhythm becomes increasingly dominated by Y (cycles 15-25). There is no phase drift, because X and Y do not interact dynamically. Note the short sleep (cycle 29) analogous to that observed in the XY model (Figure 7-1a). These short sleeps are artifacts of low Y amplitude in both models, and are not observed in real experimental data on humans. Finally, note that the period of phase-trap modulations equals that of the desynchrony beat ($\sim$ 5 cycles), due to their common origin as beat phenomena. This coincidence occurs in the model of Kronauer *et al.* (1982) for the same reason.

In all the simulations of Figure 7-1, the longest sleep episode occurs in the first beat cycle after the loss of synchrony. The phase-clustering of sleep episodes is also greatest when the simulation is just over the edge of desynchrony. Both of these observations about model behavior suggest that, for more detailed simulations of desynchrony, the models should be placed slightly beyond the synchrony/desynchrony bifurcation. When the models are too desynchronized (e.g. last 10 cycles in Figures 7-1b-d) modulation of sleep timing and duration becomes unrealistically small.

7.2 Napping and Split Sleep Simulations

None of the models discussed in Chapter 6 was designed to account for napping or split sleep patterns (Section 4.10; Sections 3.18 – 3.22). It is interesting to see how the models behave when they are pushed into this unanticipated part of parameter space.

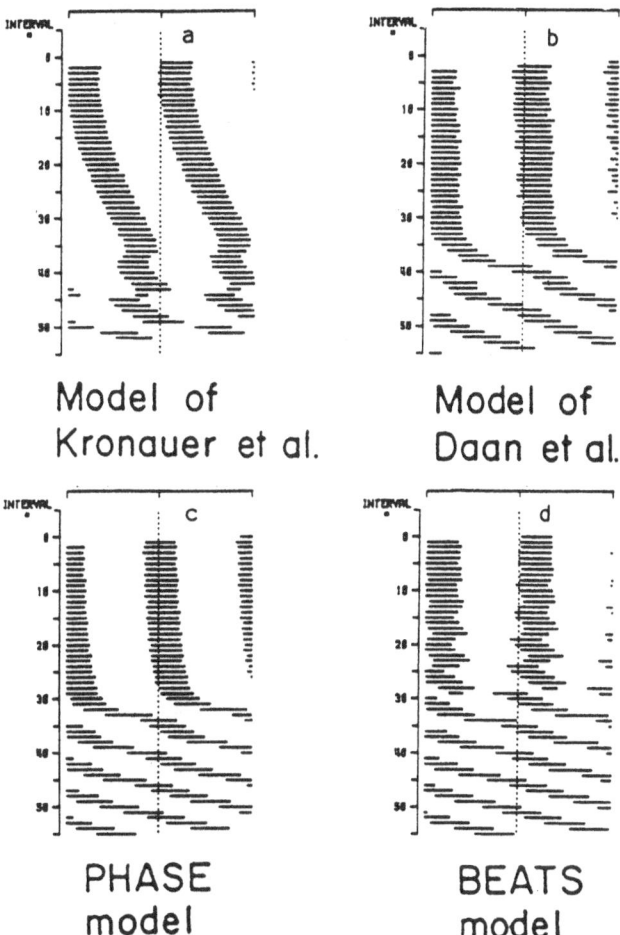

Model of
Kronauer et al.

Model of
Daan et al.

PHASE
model

BEATS
model

Figure 7-1. Transition from internal synchronization to desynchronization in 4
models of the sleep-wake cycle. All simulations were run for 50 sleep-wake
cycles, and parameters were chosen to yield an intrinsic circadian period
$\tau \sim$ 25h, intrinsic sleep-wake cycle period $\tau_{SW} \sim$ 31h, and intrinsic sleep
fraction $F \sim 0.33$. There was no feedback onto the circadian pacemaker,
except in (a), where $F_{yz} = -0.04$. The vertical midline is the locus of simulated mid-low temperature.

(a) XY model of Kronauer *et al.*, with $\hat{\tau}_y =$ 25h at the beginning of the simulation, drifting linearly to $\hat{\tau}_y =$ 31h on the last cycle. All other parameters
are standard (Section 5.3).

(b) Model of Daan *et al.*, with $\bar{H} = 0.70$, $\bar{L} = 0.06$, $p = 0.022$ and threshold
modulation amplitude A drifting linearly from 0.16 to 0.

(c) PHASE model, with dimensionless coupling k drifting linearly from $k = 2$
to 0 over the length of the simulation.

(d) BEATS model with angular threshold, and a drifts linearly from 0 to 1.
Recall that a measures the proportion of Y in the sleep-wake cycle (Section 6.2).

As a test case, I have tried to simulate napping or split sleep patterns with $\tau \sim 25$h, $\tau_{SW} \sim 14$h, and $F \sim 0.33$. A range of coupling parameters was studied for each model. The model of Kronauer *et al.* (Figure 7-2a) and the BEATS model (Figure 7-2b) fail altogether — in their present formulations they are unable to achieve any circadian modulation of sleep when τ_{SW} is as short as 14h. The PHASE model (Figure 7-2c) produces a complex sleep-wake pattern, apparently close to a 3:2 subharmonic, but not reminiscent of experimental data from humans.

The model of DAAN *et al.* generates some intriguing results (Figure 7-2d), reminiscent of both split sleep (circadian cycles 19-27) and napping (circadian cycles 33-40).

Another simulation shows in more detail the split sleep pattern predicted by the DAAN model (Figure 7-3), which at first glance resembles the record of Subject 21 in Chapter 3. Sleep is either consolidated or split into two bouts of approximately equal length. Note an unrealistic detail of the simulation: split sleep is *always* followed by a consolidated episode, whereas Subject 3.21 has two or three split episodes consecutively.

One interesting suggestion of the simulation is that split sleep, at least in the DAAN model, requires a large amplitude modulation of the threshold. We may therefore speculate why split sleep appears to be primarily a *young* person's response when asked to nap (e.g., FR20, Section 3.20): circadian rhythm amplitudes tend to decline with age (Czeisler *et al.*, 1986).

As regards napping during free-run, I have not been able to simulate the observed circadian modulation of sleep length (Sections 3.18, 3.19; 4.10). Especially elusive are the very short naps. A satisfactory model of napping remains an outstanding challenge.

7.3 A Representative Simulation of Internal Desynchrony

The aim of this section is to explore some *qualitative* aspects of the various models by comparing their simulations of one hypothetical example of desynchrony. For each model, parameters were chosen to allow simulation of a sleep-wake record with $\tau_{SW} = 34$h, $F = 0.33$, and $\tau = 25$h. There was no attempt to tailor the simulations to match any particular experimental subject; the periods and sleep fraction chosen are those of an "average" subject in the data bank of Chapter 3. All parameters were held fixed throughout the simulation so that the patterns (cf. Chapter 4) predicted by the models would not be obscured by drift.

The section begins with the models' predictions of sleep-wake raster plots. Next a variety of predicted patterns are compared to those of actual human subjects (Subjects 1, 2, 4, 10 in Chapter 3). This section considers only qualitative comparisons to data; for more quantitative evaluations, see Section 7.4.

Parameters

To simulate a hypothetical record with $\tau \sim 25$h, $\tau_{SW} = 34$h, and $F \sim 0.33$, the following parameters were selected:

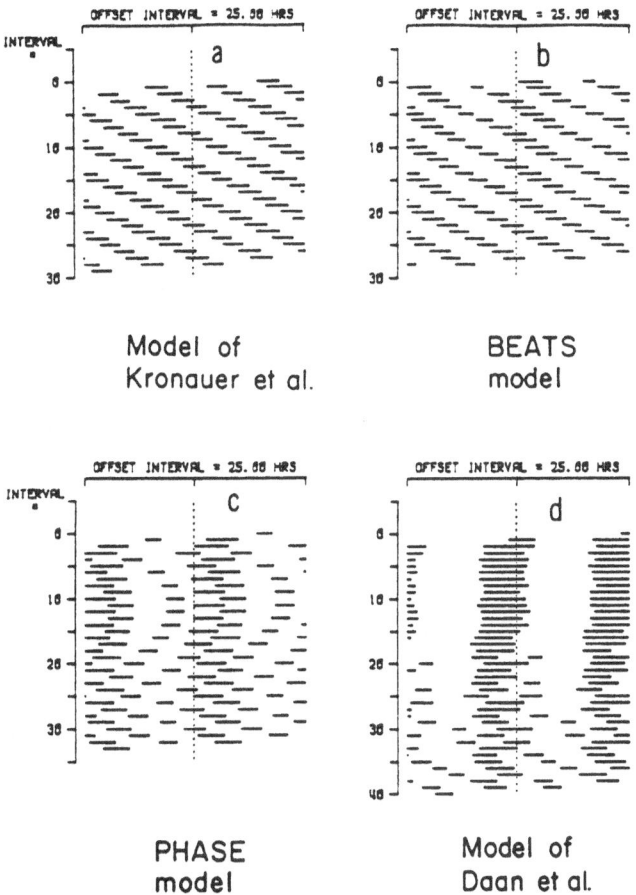

Figure 7-2. Simulations of sleep-wake patterns of free-running nappers. Each simulation is 50 sleep-wake cycles long. Vertical midline is locus of mid-low temperature. There is assumed no feedback of sleep on temperature, except in (a).

(a) XY Model of Kronauer *et al.*, with $\hat{\tau}_y = 14$h, $\hat{\tau}_z = 25$h. Couplings F_{zy} and F_{yz} are maintained at a fixed 4:1 ratio, but their absolute magnitudes decrease linearly over the simulation, from $F_{zy} = -0.24$, $F_{yz} = -0.06$ to $F_{zy} = -0.12$, $F_{yz} = -0.03$.

(b) BEATS model with angular threshold, $\tau_z = 25$, $\tau_y = 14$h. Circadian influence on sleep-wake cycle decreases linearly over simulation, beginning with $a = 0.5$, ending at $a = 0.9$.

(c) PHASE model, with $\tau_1 = 25$, $\tau_2 = 14$. Dimensionless coupling k drifts from 0.9 to 0.5.

(d) DAAN model, skewed threshold, $\bar{H} = 0.50$, $\bar{L} = 0.18$, and A drifts linearly from 0.16 to 0.06.

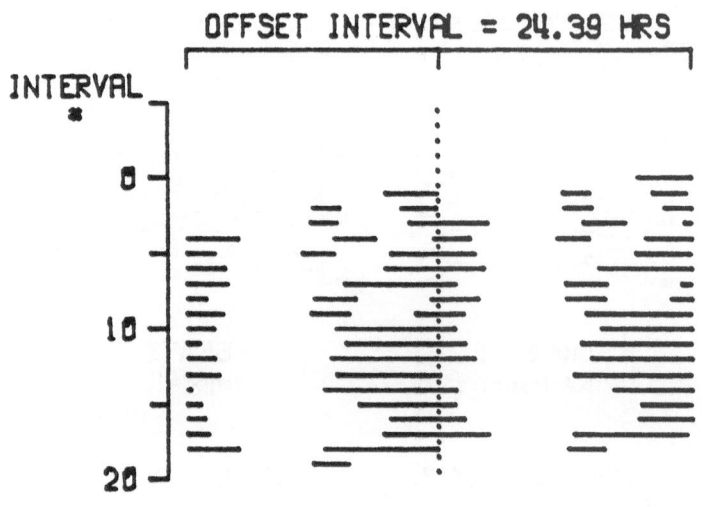

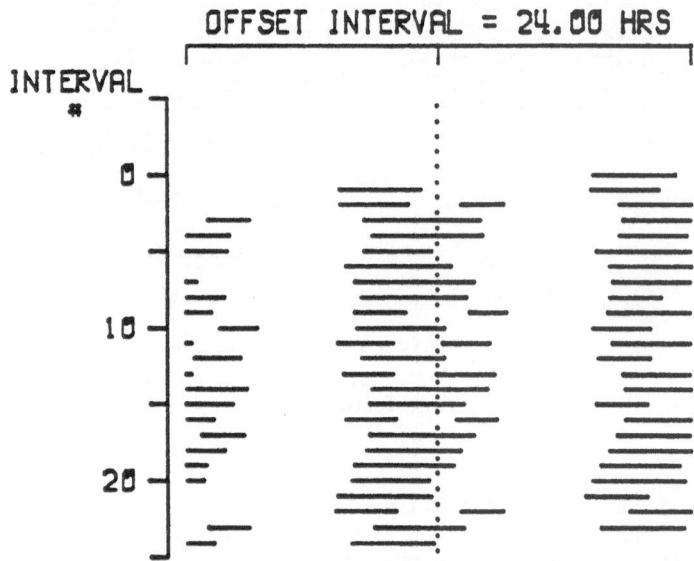

Figure 7-3. Normalized raster plots of split sleep patterns.

(top): An experimental example (Subject 3.21 of Chapter 3).

(bottom): Simulation, by modified DAAN model. Parameters were $\bar{L} = 0.18$, $\bar{H} = 0.50$, $A = 0.14$, $\tau = 24$; all other parameters set to standard values (Section 5.6).

BEATS (flat threshold): $\qquad$ $a = 0.67$, $b = 1$, $\tau_z = 25$, $\tau_y = 34$, $A_0 = -0.5$.

BEATS (angular threshold): $\qquad$ $a = 0.67$, $b = 1$, $\tau_z = 25$, $\tau_y = 34$.

PHASE: $\qquad$ $\tau_1 = 25$, $\tau_2 = 34$, $c_1 = 0$, $k = 0.8$ $(c_2 = 0.8\Omega)$.

XY (Kronauer et al., 1982) $\qquad$ $\hat{\tau}_z = 24.85$, $\hat{\tau}_y = 34$.

DAAN, SKEW with noise (Daan et al., 1984) $\qquad$ $\bar{H} = 0.74$, $\bar{L} = 0.06$, $A = 0.06$, $\tau = 25$, $p = 0.022$.

DAAN, SKEW noise = 0 (Daan et al., 1984) $\qquad$ As above, but $p = 0$.

Any parameters not mentioned above were assigned their standard values, as listed in Chapters 5 and 6.

Raster Plots

The BEATS model with the flat threshold criterion for converting Y to sleep (Section 6.2) produces some wake episodes in excess of 60h (Figure 7-4a). The cause of these unrealistic predictions was discussed near Figure 6-2. Similar problems with the flat threshold were noted by Kronauer (1982) in his interchange with Wever (1982b).

Changing the flat threshold to an angular one (Figure 7-4b) improves the BEATS model, as discussed in Section 6.2.3. There is some slight clustering of sleep onsets near low temperature, and an evident modulation of sleep length with circadian phase. In these respects the model resembles the XY model (Figure 7-4c) of Kronauer et al. (1982).

After appropriate modifications to parameters (Section 6.5) the model of Daan et al. (1984) generates the most realistic plot (Figure 7-4d). The clustering of sleep onsets is strong, and the noise in the model gives the simulation an authentic look that differs from the mathematical exactitude of the others. However, note that the noise plays an essential dynamic role in DAAN, not merely a cosmetic one; without any noise in the thresholds the model rapidly locks into an unrealistic subharmonic synchronization with the circadian cycle (Figure 7-4e).

The PHASE model (Figure 7-4f) exhibits more phase clustering than XY or BEATS, but a bit less than DAAN. That clustering is not a robust feature of the model, but merely a consequence of our choice of coupling parameter k.

Because of their completely unrealistic behavior the noiseless DAAN model and the BEATS model with the flat threshold will not be discussed in the remainder of this chapter.

Sleep Length and Circadian Phase of Sleep Onset

Section 4.1.1 addressed the relation between the length of a sleep episode (ρ) and the circadian phase (ϕ_s) at which that episode began. A number of examples of the $\phi_s{:}\rho$ relationship during internal desynchronization were shown in Chapter 3. Four of those empirical examples are reproduced in Figure 7-5 as reminders.

All the models correctly reproduce the qualitative form of the relationship (Figure 7-5). Thus the qualitative comparison to data is a weak test, failing to distinguish among models. A more rigorous version of such a test is offered in Section 7.4.

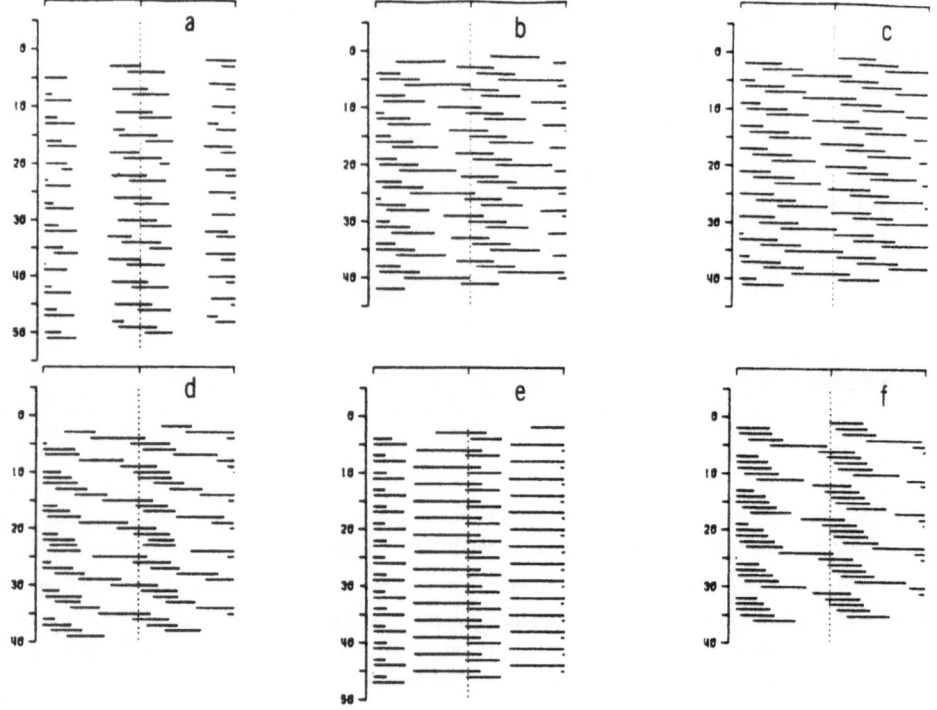

Figure 7-4. Representative simulations of an internal desynchrony (Parameters are given in the text). The rasters are normalized so that simulated mid-low temperature occurs on the dotted midline.

(a) BEATS model with flat threshold criterion.
(b) BEATS model with angular threshold.
(c) *XY* model of Kronauer *et al.*
(d) Modified model of Daan *et al.*
(e) As in (d), but without noise in the model's thresholds.
(f) PHASE model.

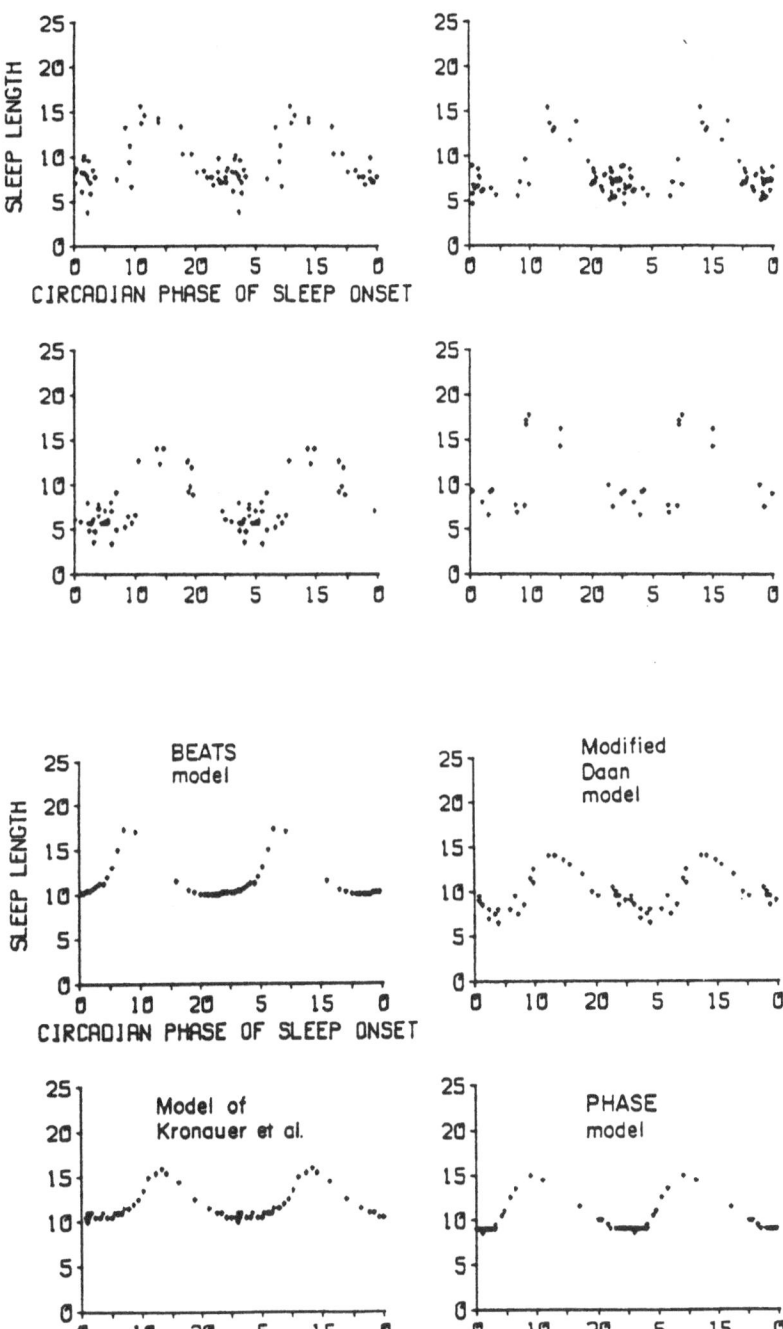

Figure 7-5. Individual examples of $\phi_s{:}\rho$ relationships, from both human subjects and model simulations. Subjects in top four panels, clockwise from upper left: 3.1, 3.2, 3.10, 3.4. See Section 7.3 for model parameters.

Phase of Sleep Onset and Length of Prior Wakefulness

There is no clear trend in the four empirical examples of Figure 7-6. Thus the overall pattern (Figure 4-1b) emerges only when data are pooled, and is not evident in individual subjects.

In contrast, the models generate unmistakably clear $\alpha{:}\phi_s$ relationships (Figure 7-6). The predicted trend is that α rises through most of the ϕ_s cycle, and decreases only in the last 5-10h before low temperature. Qualitatively, that prediction is in accord with Figure 4-1b; but a quantitative test (Section 7.4.2) reveals that *all* the models are deficient in their $\alpha{:}\phi_s$ predictions.

Sleep Length and Prior Wake Length

The pooled data from human subjects (Figures 4-2, 4-3) revealed two clouds, SHORT and LONG, in each of which α and ρ were negatively correlated. Individual subjects (Figure 7-7) show two clouds clearly enough, although the negative correlations are not always evident.

Models make interesting predictions of the $\alpha{:}\rho$ relationship in desynchrony (Figure 7-7). All except DAAN produce closed loops, with a concentration of points at short α and ρ. Notice that they do *not* predict two separate clouds, or a negative $\alpha{:}\rho$ correlation in the SHORT cloud. The DAAN model typically produces an overly large positive $\alpha{:}\rho$ correlation in desynchrony (Figure 7-7). Individual subjects conserve cycle-to-cycle sleep fraction to a lesser degree than DAAN predicts.

Wake Length and Circadian Phase of Wake-up

Section 4.9.3 emphasized that the $\phi_w{:}\alpha$ relationship in pooled data is virtually flat (Figure 4-27b). That is, knowing the circadian phase at which a wake episode begins tells us little about how long that episode will be. There is a similar finding in individual subjects (Figure 7-8). There is a weak tendency for α to shorten with increasing ϕ_w, in the range $0 \leq \phi_w \leq 10$. The longest α tend to begin after $\phi_w = 10$.

Model predictions of $\phi_w{:}\alpha$ (Figure 7-8) agree with these qualitative features. As Winfree (1983, 1984) has pointed out, the models go too far — they predict $\phi_w{:}\alpha$ relationships that are much more regular than those actually observed. This situation contrasts with that for ϕ_s and ρ (Figure 7-5) where models and data are comparably regular.

7.4 Overall Performance During Desynchrony

Each of the models is now studied over a range of parameters, corresponding to different degrees of desynchronization. Parameters controlling either the coupling of the constituent oscillators or the sleep-wake cycle period have been varied. In some cases, a desynchronization parameter has been made to increase linearly through the simulations. The results of the simulations are pooled for each model, and then compared with the empirical patterns

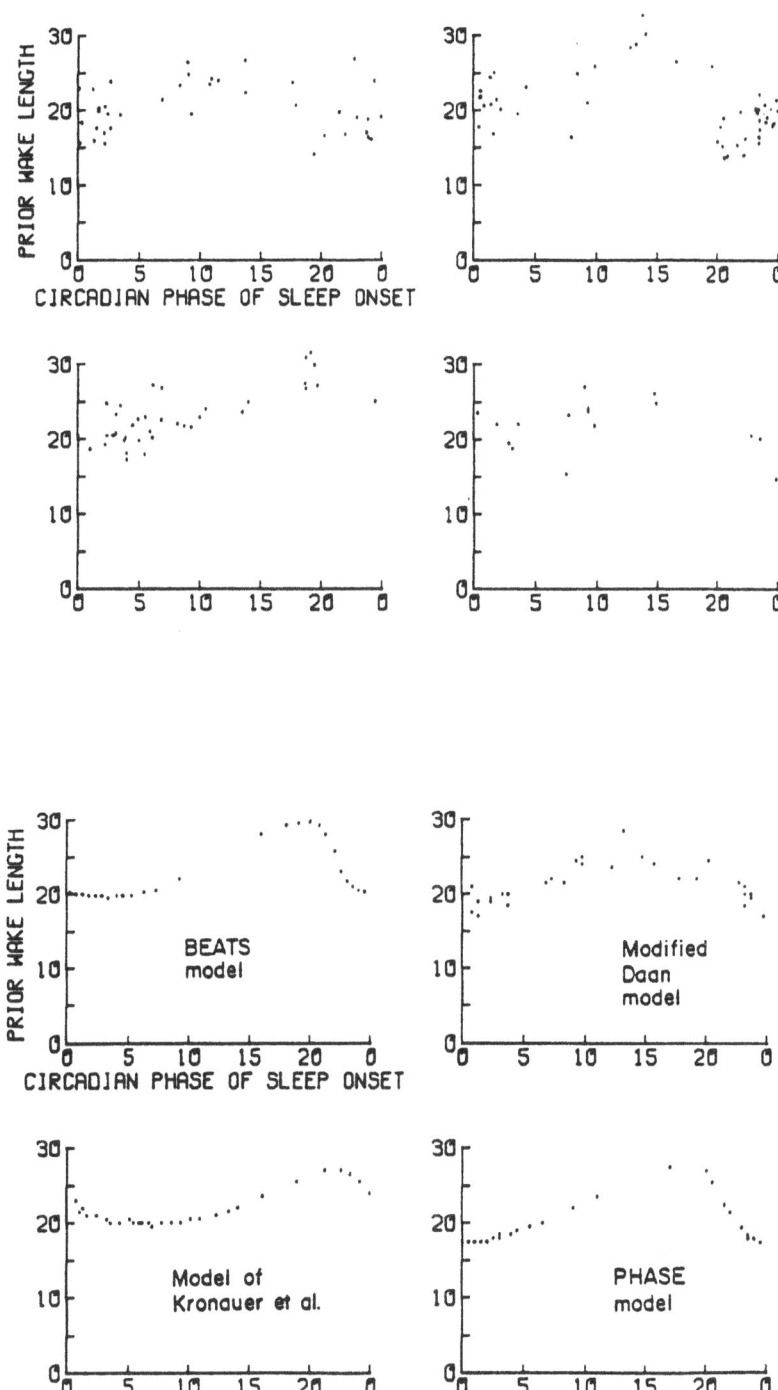

Figure 7-6. Individual examples of $\alpha{:}\phi_s$ relationships. (Format and subjects as in Figure 7-5.)

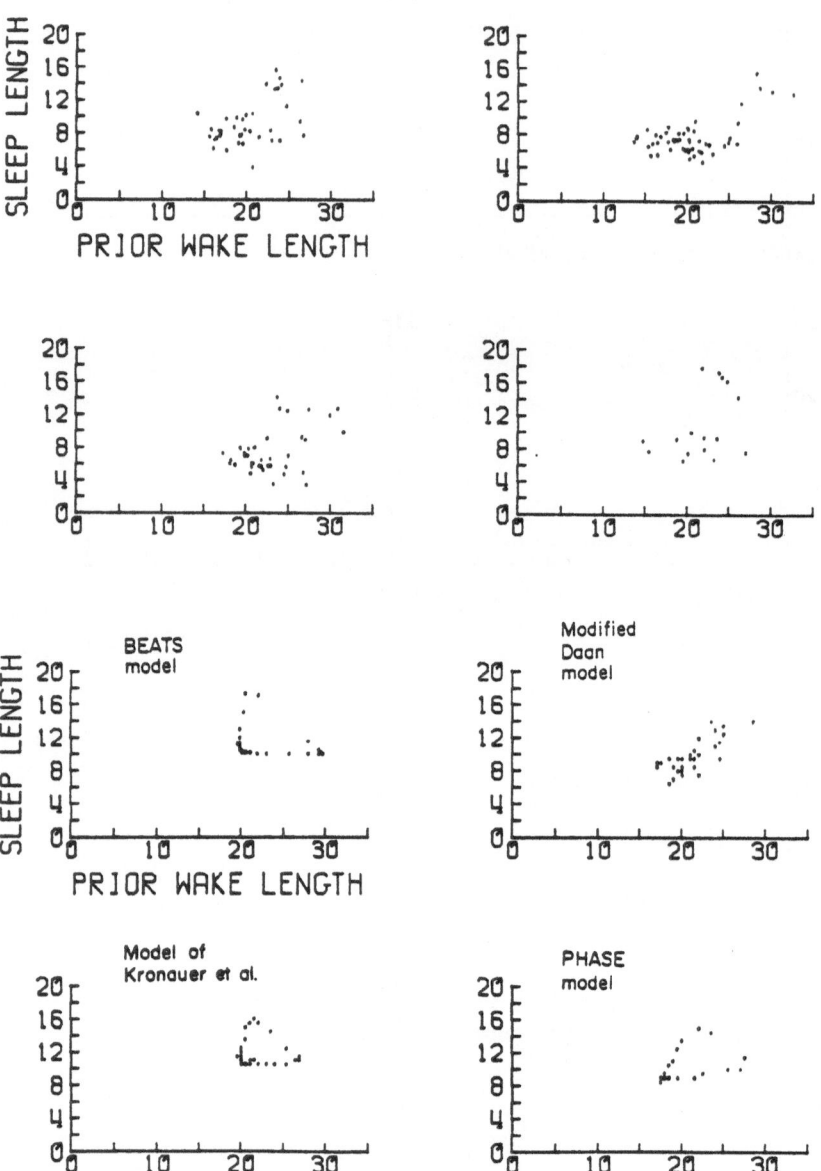

Figure 7-7. Individual examples of $\alpha{:}\rho$ relationships. (Format and subjects as in Figure 7-5.)

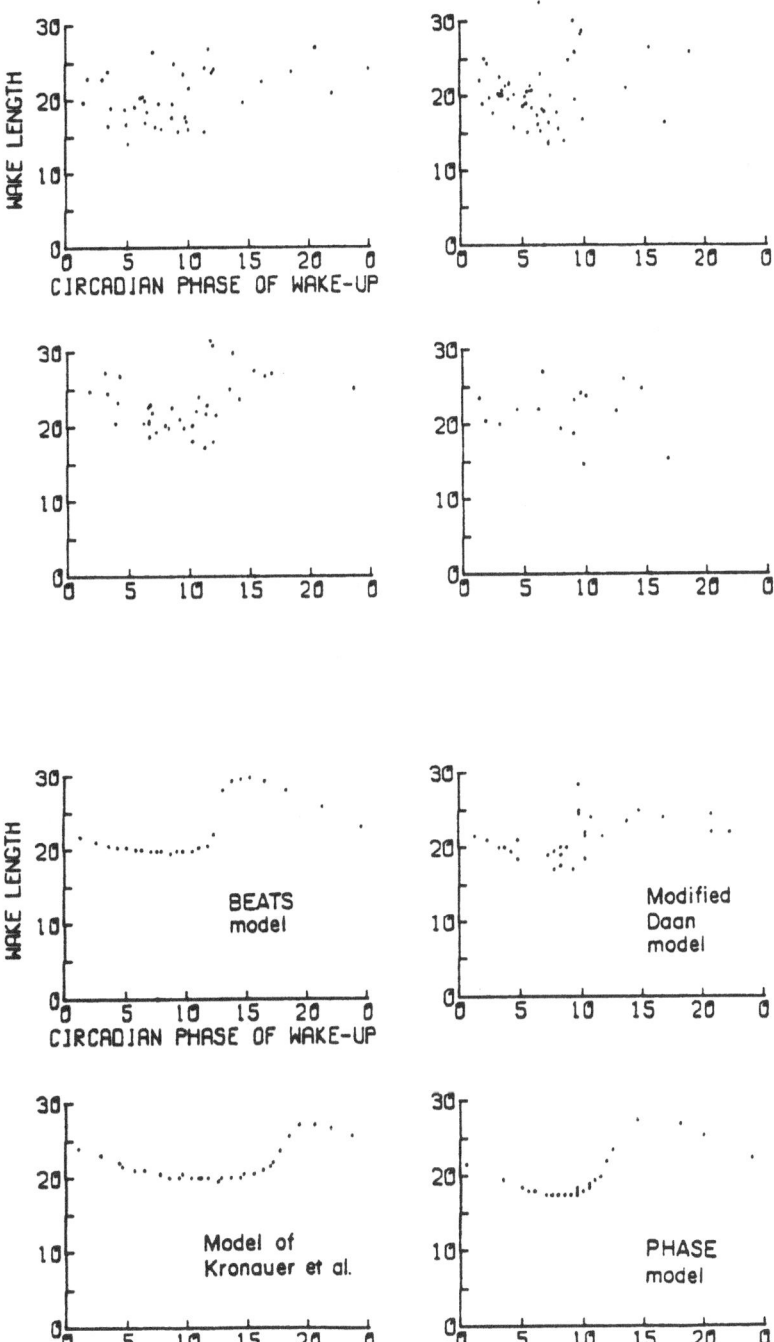

Figure 7-8. Individual examples of ϕ_w:α relationships. (Format and subjects as in Figure 7-5.)

established in Chapter 4. In this way we test the models' abilities to simulate the quantitative details of internal desynchronization.

Parameters

Table 7-1 summarizes the parameter selection. The reasons for these particular choices are now indicated briefly.

In both BEATS and PHASE, no attempt was made to fine-tune the intrinsic drive from the circadian temperature oscillator to the sleep-wake oscillator, because these models are intended to be only heuristic. A linearly drifting coupling, with secularly increasing desynchronization, allowed a more general view of these models' behaviors. Standard couplings were adopted for the models of Daan *et al.* and Kronauer *et al.*.

In all the models considered here, feedback of the sleep-wake oscillator onto the temperature oscillator affects the sleep-wake patterns very little, and was therefore ignored (except in the Kronauer XY model, where the standard feedback was adopted). The main effect of any such feedback during desynchrony is to change by $\sim 1\%$ the observed period of the temperature oscillator from its intrinsic setting. Though physiologically real (Section 4.9.1) the feedback is only a nuisance for our purposes here (for example, to give an observed τ_x of 25.0h, the parameter $\hat{\tau}_x$ had to be set near 24.85).

The intrinsic sleep-wake period was always held fixed within a simulation, but varied across simulations. The same effect was achieved for simulations of the DAAN model by altering the mean levels of the thresholds. Note that the main modifications of the DAAN model implemented here are a dramatic lowering of the wake-up threshold and a slight lowering of the sleep onset threshold (see Section 6.5.2). Compared to the original model, these changes generate higher sleep fractions and, as will be seen below, an overall better fit to many of the empirical patterns of Chapter 4.

We turn now to the models' predictions of some of those patterns.

7.4.1 Sleep Length and Circadian Phase of Sleep Onset

Figure 7-9 compares the $\phi_s{:}\rho$ relationships predicted by the models, and the pattern observed in experimental data (Section 4.1.1). The quadratic arc which was fit to the observed data has been reproduced in each panel for more direct comparison between theory and experiment.

The sleep lengths predicted by the model of Daan *et al.* (1984) are too short at all phases. No sleeps exceed 12h. This is one of the main problems of the model, given the parameters adopted by Daan *et al.* (1984). As discussed in Section 6.5.1, the difficulty was apparently overlooked while preparing the results for publication; a *superior* prediction from an earlier version of the model was accidentally substituted for the unrealistic prediction of the current model.

But the current SKEW formulation (Section 6.5) can be improved significantly by lowering the threshold levels. This modified Daan model (see Table 7-1 for parameters) agrees far better with the observed data, and actually provides the best fit of all the models considered (Figure 7-9). Its main deficiency is the omission of the vertical section of data near

Table 7-1. Model Parameters for Pooled Simulations of Internal Desynchrony

Intrinsic sleep-wake periods, and oscillator coupling constants:

BEATS:	$a = 0.55$ (beginning) $\rightarrow$ $a = 0.70$ (end); $\tau_y = 29, 31, 34.5, 38, 41.$
PHASE:	$k = 0.8 \rightarrow k = 0.5$; $\tau_2 = 29, 32, 35, 38, 41.$
XY Model of Kronauer *et al.* (1982, 1983)	$F_{xy} = -0.16$; $F_{yx} = -0.04$; $\hat{\tau}_y = 30, 32, 34, 36, 38$
Model of Daan *et al.*	$A = 0.08$; $\bar{L} = 0.16$ $H = 0.81, 0.82, 0.83, 0.84, 0.85, 0.86$
Modified Daan model	$A = 0.06$; $(\bar{L}, \bar{H}) = (0.06, 0.72),$ $(0.06, 0.74), (0.06, 0.78), (0.04, 0.75), (0.04, 0.78)$

All models:

$N = 250$ sleep episodes for BEATS, PHASE, *XY*, Modified DAAN;
$N = 270$ for DAAN
$F \sim 0.30$–0.33 (intrinsic sleep fraction parameters)
$\tau = 25.0$ (circadian period)

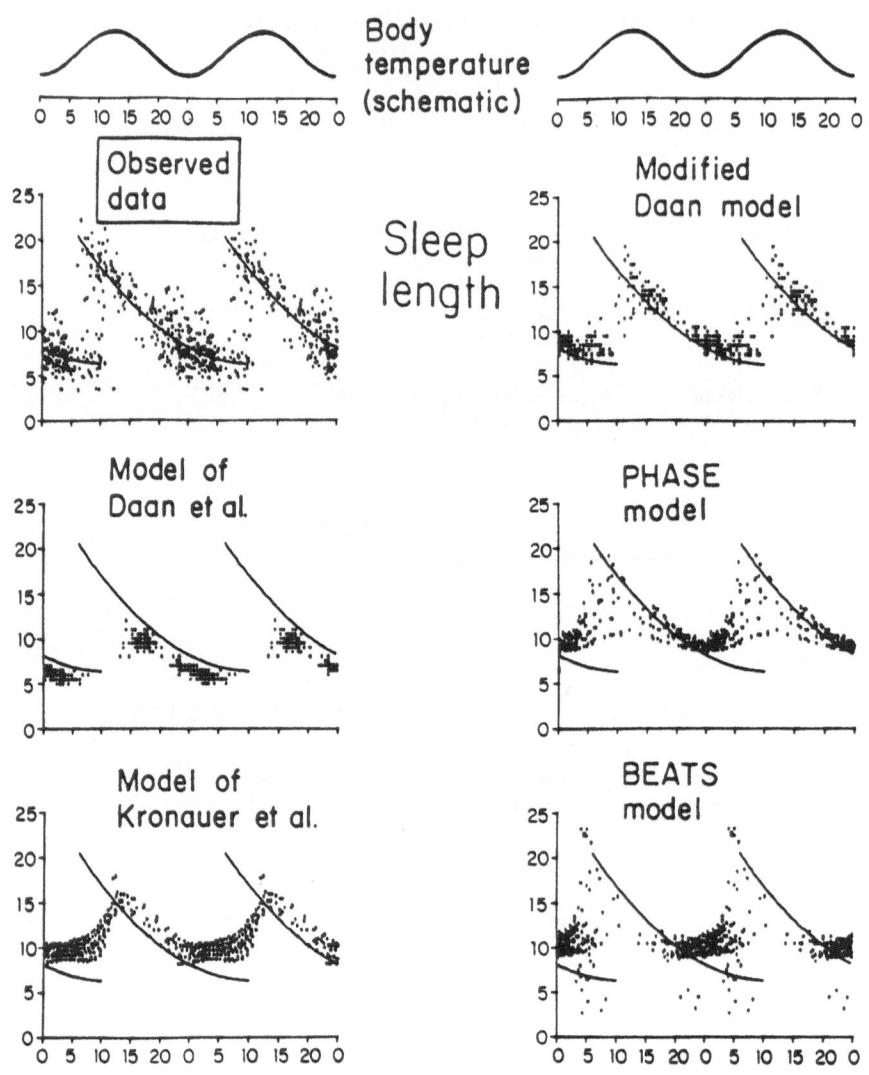

Figure 7-9. Observed and simulated scatterplots of ϕ_s:ρ relationships. Human data were pooled across Subjects 3.1 – 3.15 (see Section 4.1.1). Parameters for model simulations are listed in Table 7-1.

$\phi_s = 8-10$, and that may be a question of diddling parameters.

The XY and PHASE models each produce a striking dependence of the ϕ_s:ρ curves on the intrinsic sleep-wake cycle period. In the XY model, as $\hat{\tau}_y$ increases, the ϕ_s:ρ curve is translated upward with very little change of waveform shape, producing a visibly striated cloud in Figure 7-9. The PHASE model also produces a stack of curves parametrized by increasing τ_2, but in its case the waveforms are also sheared from sinusoidal (lowest curve) to sawtoothed (uppermost curve). This sort of shearing (Figure 5-3) as a parameter increases was anticipated qualitatively by Winfree (1983), who related it in general to the presence of a modulated threshold in a model (see Section 6.3.4 for the derivation of a modulated threshold in the PHASE model). Neither the XY model of Kronauer *et al.* nor the PHASE model correctly simulates the short sleeps occurring in $\phi_s = 0-10$. Moreover the PHASE model predicts that the ϕ_s:ρ relation is noisiest near the temperature maximum and tightest near the trough; the observed data show the opposite trend.

The BEATS model is the only one to reproduce a vertical jump between $\phi_s = 5-10$, including some very short sleeps as in the observed data. The mathematical basis for these highly variable sleep lengths is discussed in Section 6.2. The predictions are worst near the temperature trough, where ρ is almost independent of ϕ_s, instead of a decreasing function as in real data.

Conclusion: It is relatively easy to simulate the qualitative shape of the ϕ_s:ρ relation. "Long sleeps begin near high temperature, short sleeps begin near low temperature" — even models as simple as PHASE and BEATS pass the test when it is framed in this way. Such a success is therefore little cause for confidence in a model. On the other hand, when tested more rigorously against the ϕ_s:ρ data, the models reveal their deficiencies.

7.4.2. Phase of Sleep Onset and Length of Prior Wakefulness

The pooled α:ϕ_s data of Figure 4-1b (Section 4.1.2) are reproduced in Figure 7-10. Note that the data are now *single*-plotted. The data cloud has an upward slope of about 0.7, significantly less than the slope expected if all awakenings occurred at the same phase. There is a vertical section of data between $\phi_s = 18-23$.

The Daan model yields a reasonable upslope (Figure 7-10), but omits the vertical section of data. After parameter modification there is some improvement in the distribution of ϕ_s (Section 7.4.4) but not in the α:ϕ_s relation, which continues to misrepresent the vertical section of data near $\phi_s = 20$.

The XY model of Kronauer *et al.* generates a striated cloud, as in the ϕ_s:ρ relation, and the cloud becomes unrealistically slender near $\phi_s = 20$. Neither XY nor the PHASE model capture the vertical section of data, and both have insufficient maximum-to-minimum amplitude.

The BEATS model does manage a vertical data cloud near $\phi_s = 22$, but overdoes it a bit — there are some unrealistically short wakes predicted in this region.

Conclusion: None of the models reproduces the basic details of the α:ϕ_s relation. Some aspect of the control of wake duration escapes them all. The answer is not simply that wake length is influenced consciously, and hence unpredictably — such effects would more

200

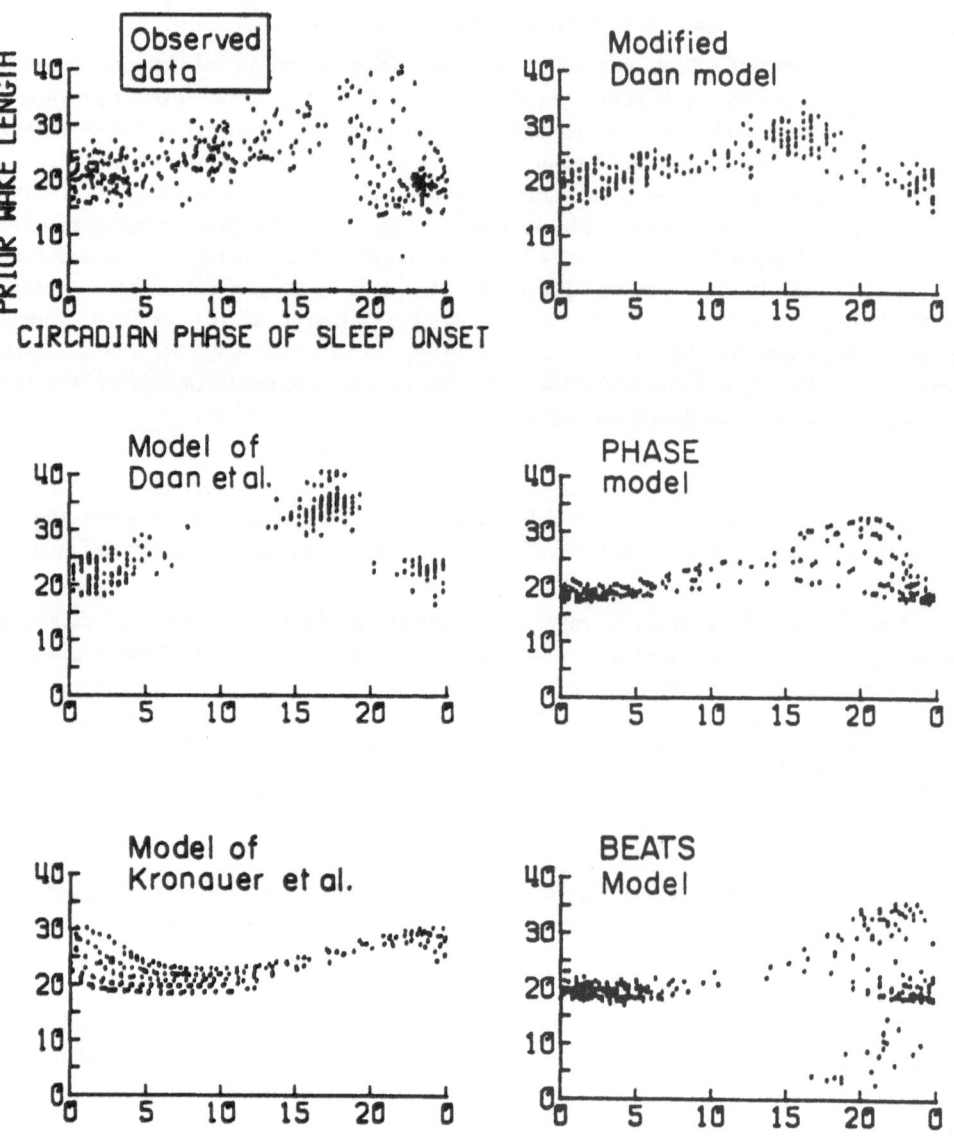

Figure 7-10. Observed and simulated $\alpha{:}\phi_s$ scatterplots. Note that the graphs are single-plotted. Format as in Figure 7-9. (See Section 4.1.2.)

likely smear the basic pattern, rather than conspire to alter it in some regular way. In other words, the data are not just noisier than the models predict; they have a different, patterned structure.

7.4.3 Phase Distribution of Wake-up

One of the findings about internal desynchronization that initially seemed most revealing was the existence of a 6h zone of "forbidden" wake-up (Winfree 1982a). It occurs just before the temperature minimum (Figure 7-11; also see Section 4.3), thereby preventing subjects from waking at a time of minimum alertness (Czeisler *et al.*, 1980a) and maximum sleep propensity (Section 4.4).

It turns out that the zone of forbidden wake-up is not difficult to simulate. As shown in Figure 7-11, the models typically generate a minimum near $\phi_w = 20$ in the distribution of spontaneous awakenings. (The model of Kronauer *et al.* is phased a few hours too late; as discussed in Section 5.3 the phase convention for defining a discrete sleep episode from the continuous y variable has been modified in the past, and perhaps the symmetric y_1, y_2 convention (Kronauer *et al.*, 1983) should be reinstated).

As regards the overall shape of the wake-up distribution, the original Daan model yields a bimodal distribution, and the Kronauer model produces a distribution with a peak frequency of only about 1.5 times the mean; both results disagree with the observations. The modified Daan model does better, but the test is not particularly demanding, as shown by the comparable success of the BEATS and PHASE models.

Conclusion: With only minor adjustment of parameters, all the models can reproduce the phase, amplitude, and unimodal shape of the wake-up distribution. The Daan model must adopt something like the modified parameters suggested in Table 7-1, while the Kronauer model needs a new phase convention for sleep, and some mechanism to increase the clustering of wake-ups.

7.4.4 Phase Distribution of Sleep Onsets

The frequency distribution of sleep onsets in the circadian cycle (Section 4.4) poses a stringent test of models. The experimentally observed distribution is bimodal, with peaks at the temperature trough and at nap phase (Figure 7-12; cf. Figures 4-7 and 4-12). The PHASE and BEATS model, and the model of Kronauer *et al.*, incorrectly predict a *unimodal* distribution. They are unable to account for the nap phase peak, a deficiency which is not too surprising given that all three models lack a prominent "second harmonic" component. The Daan model generates a bimodal distribution, but its amplitude is excessive (sleep onsets too clustered) and its nap phase peak is about 8h too late. The modified Daan model improves the distribution's amplitude but not the phasing of the nap peak.

Conclusion: The models considered here should be viewed skeptically, with regard to their predictions of the timing of sleep onset during internal desynchronization. The modified Daan model is most successful, but its upper threshold must be reshaped *ad hoc* in order to produce a truly realistic fit to the data.

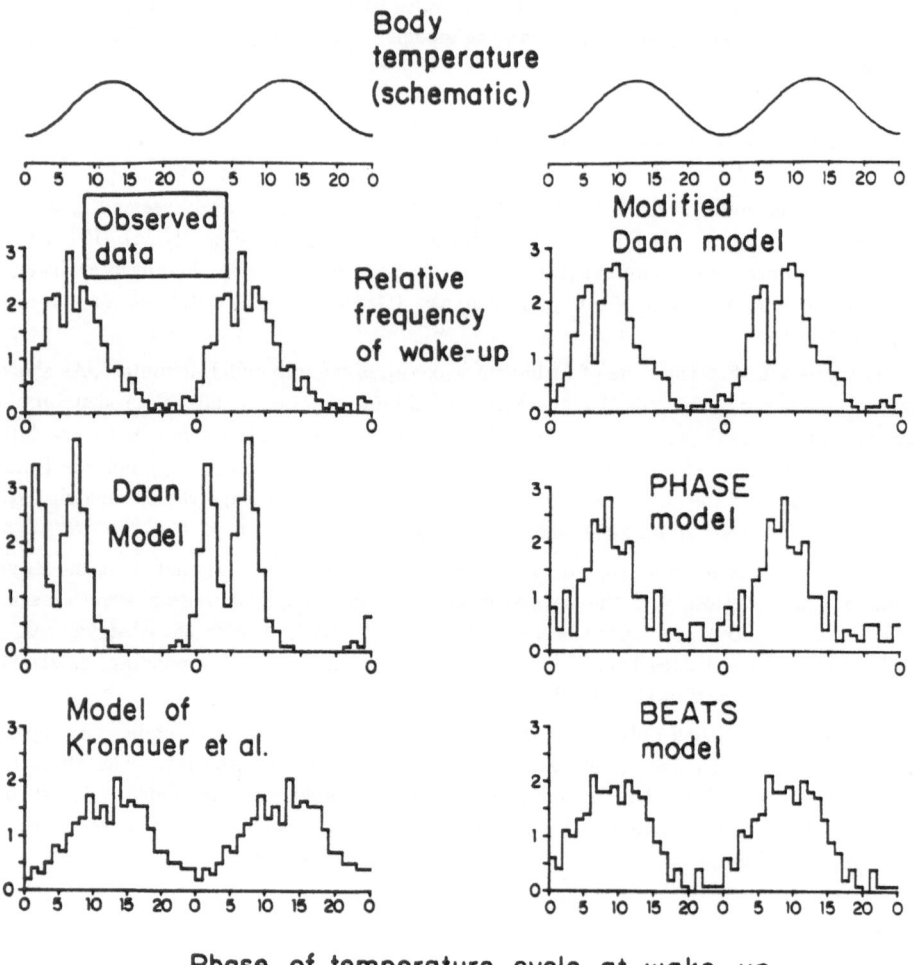

Figure 7-11. Observed and simulated distributions of wake-ups in the circadian cycle. Format as in Figure 7-9. (See Section 4.3.)

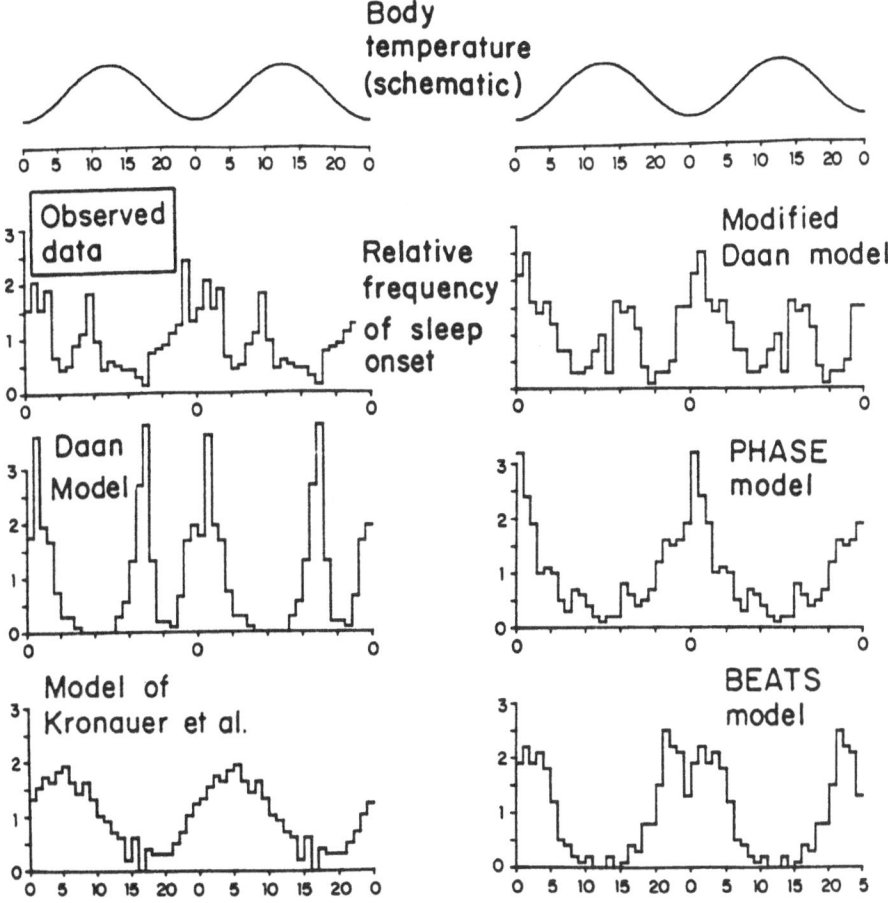

Phase of temperature cycle at sleep onset

Figure 7-12. Observed and simulated distributions of bedtimes in the circadian cycle. Format as in Figure 7-9. (See Section 4.4.)

7.4.5 Sleep Length and Prior Wake Length

The pooled $\alpha{:}\rho$ data (Figure 4-2) are reproduced in Figure 7-13. The diagonally sloping clouds of the actual data are not well captured by the XY, PHASE, or BEATS models. The DAAN model generates two clouds but with insufficiently negative $\alpha{:}\rho$ correlation (Section 4.2) within each cloud. The $\alpha{:}\rho$ scatterplot predicted by the modified Daan model lacks the variability of the observed data but otherwise its resemblance is good.

Conclusion: As in Section 7.4.4, the modified Daan model performs better than the controls (PHASE and BEATS) and the XY and DAAN models.

7.4.6 Wake Length and Phase of Wake-up

As discussed in Section 4.9.3, the $\phi_w{:}\alpha$ relationship (Figure 7-14) provides a sharp test of models. The large variability of wake durations observed for episodes beginning in the first half of the circadian cycle is not predicted successfully by the XY, PHASE, or BEATS models. In this respect the XY model is not superior to the controls. The DAAN model predicts a double-valued distribution of wake length that is overly well defined, a problem remedied to a large extent in the modified model.

Conclusion: With regard to matching the $\phi_w{:}\alpha$ data, the modified Daan model is superior to the controls, while the DAAN and XY models are not.

7.5 Summary and Discussion

7.5.1 Summary

The results of Section 7.1 concern the transition from internal synchrony to desynchrony in the DAAN, XY, PHASE, and BEATS models. The BEATS and XY models phase-trap before desynchrony occurs, whereas the PHASE and DAAN models do not. In all four models, realistic simulations of desynchrony require the system to be placed just over the "edge" — parameters corresponding to more extreme desynchronization produce an unrealistically small modulation of sleep timing and duration.

None of the models accounts for napping (Section 7.2), although the DAAN model can generate simulations reminiscent of split sleep patterns (Section 4.10).

Sections 7.3 and 7.4 address simulations of the patterns characteristic of internal desynchrony (Chapter 4). On qualitative comparisons between human data and simulated raster plots (Figure 7-4) or individual $\phi_s{:}\rho$ plots (Figure 7-5), the DAAN and XY models do not outperform the simpler control models PHASE and BEATS. Nor do the $\alpha{:}\phi_s$ (Figure 7-6), $\alpha{:}\rho$ (Figure 7-7), and $\phi_w{:}\alpha$ (Figure 7-8) plots for *individual* simulations discriminate decisively among models.

Much stronger tests are afforded by comparing *pooled* simulation results against *pooled* data (Section 7.4). The control models simulate the $\phi_s{:}\rho$ (Figure 7-9) and ϕ_w distribution data (Figure 7-11) about as well as the XY and DAAN models. However, a modified version of the model of Daan *et al.* (1984), containing a lowered threshold for wake-up, is

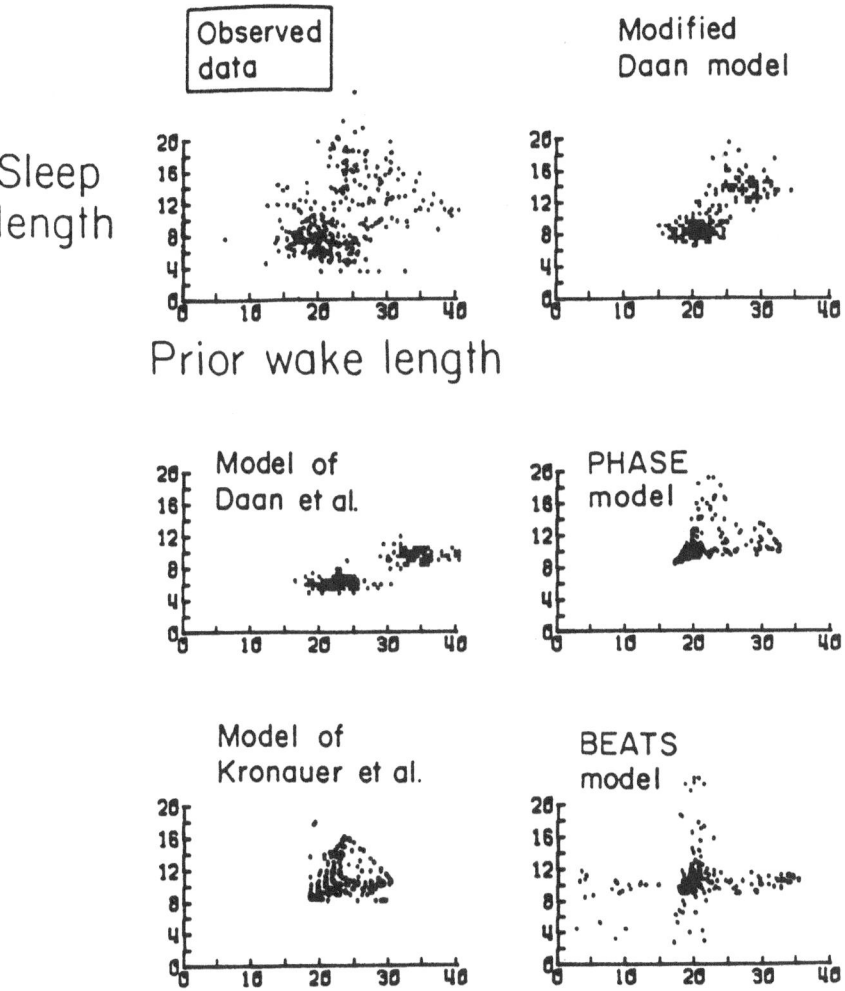

Figure 7-13. Observed and simulated $\alpha{:}\rho$ scatterplots. (See Section 4.2)

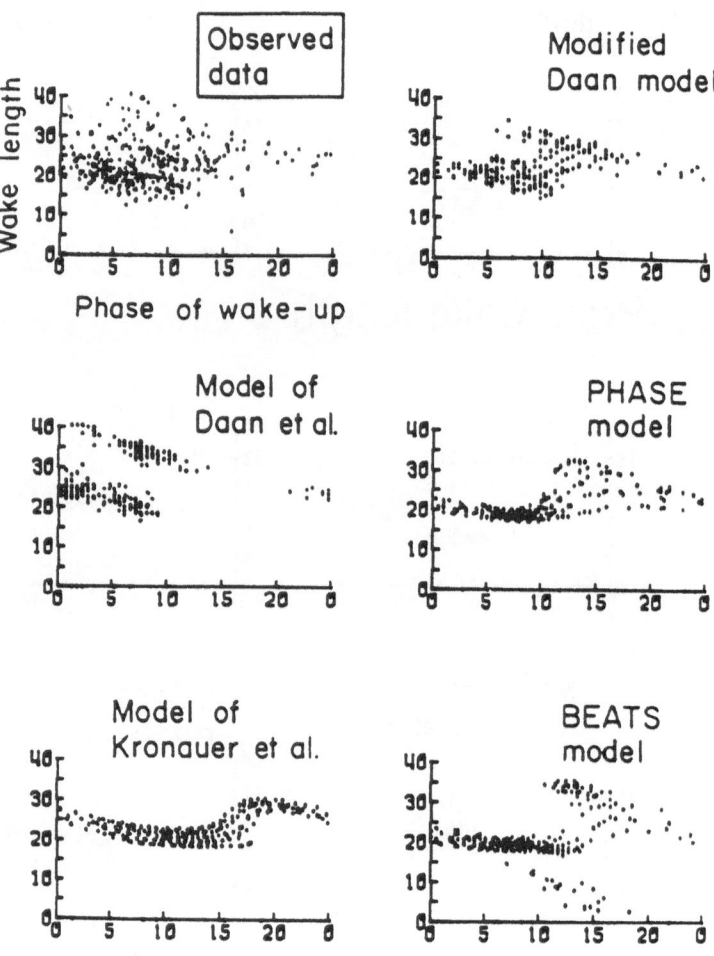

Figure 7-14. Observed and simulated $\phi_w{:}\alpha$ scatterplots. (See Section 4.9.3)

superior to the controls *and* the XY and DAAN models, when tested against the ϕ_s distribution (Figure 7-12), the α:ρ plot (Figure 7-13) and the ϕ_w:α plot (Figure 7-14).

In summary: with regard to simulations of data from internally desynchronized free-run, only the modified Daan model performs consistently better than the control models. Yet even it does not provide a quantitative match to data.

7.5.2 Discussion

Both the models of Kronauer *et al.* (1982, 1983) and Daan *et al.* (1984; Daan and Beersma, 1984) have influenced much of the current thinking about the human sleep-wake cycle. The main finding of this chapter is that neither of these models is significantly more accurate than the control models PHASE and BEATS, with respect to simulations of internally desynchronized free-run. However, a modified version of the DAAN model produces a superior fit to the desynchrony data.

It is important to understand the limitations of this result. Throughout the present study, internal desynchrony has been selected as the sole arena for competition between the models, first because so much quantitative experimental data is available about this phenomenon, and second, because it is the only sleep-wake phenomenon which *both* the Daan and Kronauer groups have addressed *in detail*. Yet other phenomena deserve comparable attention.

For example, Kronauer and colleagues have considered a number of very interesting and practical problems about entrainment to zeitgebers (Kronauer, 1984; Gander *et al.*, 1984a,b, 1985; Moore-Ede *et al.*, 1986), whereas Daan *et al.* (1984) prefer to postpone such attempts until the resetting effects of light and other zeitgebers are better characterized in humans. On similar grounds, Daan *et al.* (1984) choose not to address the consistent finding that the circadian temperature cycle shortens when the sleep-wake cycle desynchronizes from it (Section 4.9.3).

On the other hand, the XY model is essentially silent about the relation between the y-process and the internal organization of sleep, whereas the S-process of Daan *et al.* (1984) is closely tied to the observed EEG characteristics of slow-wave sleep. The S-process also accounts neatly for certain results of sleep deprivation experiments (Borbely, 1982).

Therefore the natural question — "Which is the best available model of the human circadian system?" has no easy answer at the present time. In general, the XY model offers the better account of the *circadian cycle* and the changes in its timing induced by altered sleep-wake and entrainment schedules, whereas the DAAN model more successfully describes the timing and internal structure of *sleep*. Because their strengths are complementary, it may be possible to formulate a hybrid which incorporates the best features of both models.

Chapter 8

Epilogue

This final chapter reviews the main contributions of the monograph, and suggests some possible directions for future research.

8.1 Contributions

A Data Bank of Internal Desynchronization

A number of sleep-wake records have been collected, standardized, and reanalyzed in Chapter 3. They were drawn from experiments conducted by groups in France, Germany, the United Kingdom, and the United States. No such collection and synthesis has ever appeared before.

In the past, these records have either been scattered in journals, books, government reports, or else they have never been published. Hence there has been considerable uncertainty about the general properties of sleep-wake timing during internal desynchronization. Much previous theorizing has relied on the same few experimental examples again and again, with no guarantee that these examples are representative. The data assembled here provide a starting point for sounder assessments of both the diversity and the unity of desynchronized sleep-wake patterns.

Extraction of Empirical Regularities

The individual sleep-wake records of Chapter 3 have been pooled, reanalyzed, and replotted to distill their common structural features. The key findings are summarized in Section 4.11. One family of results underscores the importance of the timing of sleep onset relative to the circadian cycle: the circadian phase of sleep onset determines the durations of the subsequent sleep episode, the prior wake episode, and the wake-sleep cycle. These findings illuminate the subtle dependence of sleep length (ρ) on prior wake length (α), a controversial topic in the past. Moreover, the circadian dependence of α and ρ reconciles the seemingly contradictory $\alpha{:}\rho$ correlations observed during synchronized and desynchronized free-run, and refutes an intuitively plausible restorative model of sleep duration. The frequency distributions of self-selected sleep and wake onsets in the circadian cycle reveal an important asymmetry: wake-ups are distributed unimodally, but bedtimes are distributed bimodally, with a secondary peak corresponding to the time of afternoon napping. This finding suggests an innate nap tendency in man. Bracketing the nap phase are two valleys in the sleep onset distribution — the "wake-maintenance zones." During one of these zones, about 8 hours before the minimum of the circadian temperature cycle, subjects consistently found it difficult to fall asleep, even in such disparate conditions as high frequency sleep schedules and entrainment to non-24 hour day lengths. This most important finding links circadian phase dysfunction to certain types of insomnia. Finally, two previously proposed regularities — phase-trapping and the secular lengthening of the sleep-wake cycle — are reviewed critically, and the properties of free-running nap and split sleep patterns are presented. Taken together, the results of Chapter 4 provide much new and fundamental information about the intrinsic dynamics of the human sleep-wake cycle.

Comparative Analysis of Models

Whereas the first four chapters concern empirical questions, the last three chapters focus on mathematical models of the sleep-wake cycle. Recently, this has been an exciting area of research, characterized by vigorous denunciation of the other fellow's model and defense of one's own. For example, see the exchange between Kronauer (1982) and Wever (1982b), as well as that between Daan et al. (1984) and Kronauer and Gander (1984). To resolve some of the issues raised by these and other modelers, I have assembled the facts about internal desynchronization, a body of data which all agree must be accounted for by any viable model. The present work is the first to simulate each of the various models and to test them against the same data base.

Moreover, to gain perspective about model performance, two simple models have been developed as "controls" (Sections 6.2, 6.3). In qualitative respects, these simple models fit the data from internal desynchrony as well as the more sophisticated models of Daan et al. (1984) and Kronauer et al. (1982), suggesting that such successes are not as impressive as they might appear (Chapter 7). However, with some modifications proposed here, the model of Daan et al. outperforms the control models. On more discriminating tests all of the models fall short.

In addition to serving as controls, the two models introduced here are the first analytically tractable models of the sleep-wake cycle. Graphical solution of their governing equations elucidates the numerically predicted interrelations among sleep length, prior wake length, circadian phase, etc. Furthermore, phase plane analyses demonstrate some unexpected connections among the simple models and the models of Daan et al. (1984) and Kronauer et al. (1982).

Thus the findings presented in Chapters 6 and 7 synthesize the work of several theorists, and provide a rational framework for comparing models against one another.

8.2 Directions for Future Research

Experimental Directions

Given the pervasive influence of the circadian pacemaker on the sleep-wake cycle, it is the first order of business to develop accurate, rapid, and inexpensive assays of circadian phase. In other words, on a given day, when does some reference point in the circadian cycle occur? The usual reference is the minimum of body temperature, but it is easily masked by changes in activity, posture, emotional state, etc. The "constant routine" protocol of Czeisler et al. (1985, 1986) is an important step in the right direction (see Section 4.5.3). By keeping posture, feeding, activity, and lighting constant, this routine exposes more nearly the "endogenous" waveform of body temperature. Unfortunately it requires the subject to be sleep-deprived for 40-70h, an intervention which may itself shift the clock.

With an assay for circadian phase in hand, a number of crucial questions become amenable to investigation. How does light shift the circadian clock? Circadian phase assessments before and after intervention with bright light could help determine the phase resetting properties of the human circadian system. Is sleep itself capable of phase-shifting the circadian pacemaker? The approach here might be to displace sleep, as in a simulated jet lag study, while keeping the ambient light intensity below the phase-shifting threshold presumably determined in the first set of experiments. (Dim light is required to avoid confounding the effects of displaced sleep.) The phase-resetting effects of both light and sleep must be understood before we can devise rational approaches to shift work scheduling and the treatment of jet lag.

A question of methodological importance concerns the free-run protocol itself, and the role of volition in internal desynchrony. What are the consequences of the usual experimental instructions to avoid naps? Is internal desynchrony somehow induced by adherence to these instructions? (See Section 4.9.3.) How do the traditional free-run results compare with those obtained under different unscheduled protocols, such as Campbell's (1984) "disentrainment", in which subjects are forbidden to structure their day around meals, mental diversions, or anything else?

Theoretical Directions

First of all, what can one reasonably hope to gain by mathematical modeling at this time? As such modeling remains necessarily phenomenological, it seems overly optimistic to expect quantitative accuracy in predictions of *sleep-wake* behavior. Indeed none of the models examined is particularly successful in this regard. However, as distinct from sleep, the response of the *circadian pacemaker* to various schedules and lighting regimes is perhaps more easily modeled, and is probably more important for applications to shift work, jet lag, and sleep-scheduling disorders. The model of Kronauer *et al.* (1982; Gander *et al.*, 1984a,b) is currently the only one to address this issue. Once the feedback of light and sleep on the circadian system is characterized, other such models will be developed.

The models available today are at their best when they help us to distinguish between experimental findings which follow from general mathematical considerations, as opposed to those which require special biological explanations. For example, almost any reasonable model can correctly predict the shape of the relationship between sleep length and circadian phase (Section 7.4.1) — the relationship emerges as a general consequence of circadian modulation of the sleep-wake cycle. In contrast, the existence of the nap phase (Section 4.4), the evening wake-maintenance zone (Section 4.5) and anomalous circadian phases during entrainment (Section 3.9), are all beyond the reach of current models, indicating that some important biology is missing from them.

The next step in theoretical sleep research may be the incorporation of sleep stages, including the interaction between the circadian cycle and REM sleep. Some initial efforts have already been made (Borbély, 1982; McCarley and Massaquoi, 1983). There are some intriguing mysteries here regarding the possible competition between slow-wave sleep and REM sleep (Carskadon and Dement, 1977), with implications for the pathophysiology and treatment of some types of depression (Wehr and Goodwin, 1983; Beersma *et al.*, 1984).

REFERENCES

Åkerstedt, T. and Fröberg, J.E. (1977). Psychophysiological circadian rhythms in women during 72h of sleep deprivation, *Waking and Sleeping* 1, 387–394.

Åkerstedt, T. and Gillberg, M. (1981). The circadian variation of experimentally displaced sleep, *Sleep* 4 (2), 159–169.

Aschoff, J. (1965). Circadian rhythms in man, *Science* 148, 1427–1432.

Aschoff, J. (1969). Desynchronization and resynchronization of human circadian rhythms, *Aerospace Medicine* 40, 844–849.

Aschoff, J., ed. (1981). *Handbook of Behavioral Neurobiology*, Vol. 4: *Biological Rhythms*, (Plenum Press, New York).

Aschoff, J. and Wever, R. (1962). Spontanperiodik des Menschen bei Ausschluss aller Zeitgeber, *Naturwissenschaften* 49, 337–342.

Aschoff, J., Gerecke, U. and Wever, R. (1967). Desynchronization of human circadian rhythms, *Japanese J. Physiol.* 17, 450–457.

Aschoff, J., Gerecke, U., Kureck, A., Pohl, H., Rieger, P., von Saint-Paul, U., and Wever, R. (1971), Interdependent parameters of circadian activity rhythms in birds and man, in: *Biochronometry*, vol. 3, ed. M. Menaker (National Acad. of Sciences, Washington, D.C.), pp. 3-27.

Aschoff, J. and Wever, R. (1976). Human circadian rhythms: A multioscillatory system, *Fed. Proc.* 35, 2326–2332.

Aschoff, J. and Wever, R. (1981). The circadian system of man, in: *Handbook of Behavioral Neurobiology*, Vol. 4: *Biological Rhythms*, ed. J. Aschoff (Plenum Press, New York), pp. 311-331.

Aschoff, J., Wever, R., Wildgruber, C., and Wirz-Justice, A. (1984). Circadian control of meal timing during temporal isolation, *Naturwissenschaften* 71, 534–535.

Beersma, D.G.M., Daan, S., Hoofdakker, R.H. Van Den (1984). Distribution of REM latencies and other sleep phenomena in depression as explained by a single ultradian rhythm disturbance, *Sleep* 7 (2), 126–136.

Borbély, A.A. (1982). A two process model of sleep regulation, *Human Neurobiology* 1, 195-204.

Borbély, A.A. and Tobler, I. (1980). The search for an endogenous "sleep-substance", *Trends Pharmacol.* 1, 356–358.

Borbély, A.A:, Baumann, F., Brandeis, D., Strauch, I., and Lehman, D. (1981). Sleep deprivation: Effect on sleep stages and EEG power density in man, *Electroencephalogr. Clin. Neurophysiol.* 51, 483–493.

Broughton, R. (1975). Biorhythmic variations in consciousness and psychological functions, *Can. Psychol. Rev.* 16, 217–239.

Broughton, R. (Symposium Chairman) (1983). The siesta: Social or biological phenomenon? *Sleep Res.* 12, 28–30.

Campbell, S.S. (1984). Duration and placement of sleep in a "disentrained" environment, *Psychophysiology* **21**, 106–113.

Carpenter, G.A. and Grossberg, S. (1983). A neural theory of circadian rhythms: The gated pacemaker, *Biol. Cybern.* **48**, 35–59.

Carpenter, G.A. and Grossberg, S. (1984). A neural theory of circadian rhythms: Aschoff's rule in diurnal and nocturnal mammals, *Am. J. Physiol.* **247**, R1067–R1082.

Carskadon, M.A. (1985). MSLT and unintentional sleep episodes on a constant routine, pre-print.

Carskadon, M.A. and Dement, W.C. (1975). Sleep studies on a 90-minute day, *Electroencephalogr. Clin. Neurophysiol.* **39**, 145–155.

Carskadon, M.A. and Dement, W.C. (1977). Sleepiness and sleep state on a 90-min. schedule, *Psychophysiology* **14**, 127–133.

Carskadon, M.A. and Dement, W.C. (1980). Distribution of REM sleep on a 90-minute sleep-wake schedule, *Sleep* **2**, 309–317.

Carskadon, M.A. and Dement, W.C. (1985). Midafternoon decline in MSLT scores on a constant routine, *Sleep Res.* **14**, 292.

Chouvet, G., Mouret, J., Coindet, J., Siffre, M., and Jouvet, M. (1974). Periodicité bicircadienne du cycle vielle-sommeil dans des conditions hors du temps, *Electroencephalogr. Clin. Neurophysiol.* **37**, 367–380.

Cohen, A.H., Holmes, P.J., and Rand, R.H. (1982). The nature of the coupling between segmental oscillators of the lamprey spinal generator for locomotion: A mathematical model, *J. Math. Biol.* **13**, 345–369.

Colquhoun, W.P., ed. (1971). *Biological Rhythms and Human Performance*, (Academic Press, London).

Colquhoun, W.P., ed. (1972). *Aspects of Human Efficiency*, (English Univ. Press, London).

Czeisler, C.A. (1978). Human circadian physiology: Internal organization of temperature, sleep-wake and neuroendocrine rhythms monitored in an environment free of time-cues, Ph.D. Thesis, Stanford University, Stanford, CA.

Czeisler, C.A., Weitzman, E.D., Moore-Ede, M.C., Zimmerman, J.C., and Knauer, R.S. (1980a). Human sleep: Its duration and organization depend on its circadian phase, *Science* **210**, 1264–1267.

Czeisler, C.A., Zimmerman, J.C., Ronda, J.M., Moore-Ede, M.C., and Weitzman, E.D. (1980b). Timing of REM sleep is coupled to the circadian rhythm of body temperature in man, *Sleep* **2**, 329–346.

Czeisler, C.A., Richardson, G.S., Coleman, R.M., Zimmerman, J.C., Moore-Ede, M.C., Dement, W.C., and Weitzman, E.D. (1981). Chronotherapy: Resetting the circadian clocks of patients with delayed sleep phase insomnia, *Sleep* **4** (1), 1–21.

Czeisler, C.A., Moore-Ede, M.C., and Coleman, R.M. (1982). Rotating shift work schedules that disrupt sleep are improved by applying circadian principles, *Science* **217**, 460–463.

Czeisler, C.A., Brown, E.N., Ronda, J.M., Kronauer, R.E., Richardson, G.S. and Freitag, W.O. (1985). A clinical method to assess the endogenous circadian phase (ECP) of the deep circadian oscillator in man, *Sleep Res.* **14**, 295.

Czeisler, C.A., Rios, C.D., Brown, E.N., Richardson, G.S., Ronda, J.M., Rogacz, S., and Williams, G.H. (1986). A clinical method to assess the phase of the endogenous circadian oscillator in man, preprint.

Daan, S. and Berde, C. (1978). Two coupled oscillators: Simulations of the circadian pacemaker in mammalian activity rhythms, *J. Theor. Biol.* **70**, 297–313.

Daan, S. and Beersma, D. (1984). Circadian gating of human sleep-wake cycles, in: *Mathematical Models of the Circadian Sleep-Wake Cycle*, eds. M.C. Moore-Ede and C.A. Czeisler, (Raven Press, New York), pp. 129–158.

Daan, S., Beersma, D.G.M., and Borbély, A.A. (1984). Timing of human sleep: Recovery process gated by a circadian pacemaker, *Am. J. Physiol.* **246**, R161-R178.

Dirlich, G. (1984). Looking at human circadian phenomena from a framework of simple stochastic models, in: *Mathematical Models of the Circadian Sleep-Wake Cycle*, eds. M.C. Moore-Ede and C.A. Czeisler, (Raven Press, New York), pp. 159–186.

Dorrscheidt, G.J and Beck, L. (1975). Advanced methods for evaluating characteristic parameters (τ, α, ρ) of circadian rhythms, *J. Math. Biol.* **2**, 107–121.

Eastman, C. (1984). Are separate temperature and activity oscillators necessary to explain the phenomena of human circadian rhythms? In: *Mathematical Models of the Circadian Sleep-Wake Cycle*, eds. M.C. Moore-Ede and C.A. Czeisler, (Raven Press, New York), pp. 81–103.

Elliott, A.L., Mills, J.N., and Waterhouse, J.M. (1971). A man with too long a day, *J. Physiol.* (London) **212**, 30–31P.

Enright, J.T. (1980). *The Timing of Sleep and Wakefulness*, Studies in Brain Function, **3**, (Springer-Verlag, Berlin).

Enright, J.T. (1984). Sleep duration for human subjects during internal desynchronization, in: *Mathematical Models of the Circadian Sleep-Wake Cycle*, eds. M.C. Moore-Ede and C.A. Czeisler, (Raven Press, New York), pp. 201–205.

Ermentrout, G.B. and Kopell, N. (1984). Frequency plateaus in a chain of weakly coupled oscillators, I, *SIAM J. Math. Anal.* **15**, 215–237.

Ermentrout, G.B. and Rinzel, J. (1984). Beyond a pacemaker's entrainment limit: Phase walk-through, *Am. J. Physiol.* **246**, R102-R106.

Fookson, J.E., Kronauer, R.E., Weitzman, E.D., Monk, T.H., Moline, M.L., and Hoey, E. (1984). Induction of insomnia on non-24 hour sleep-wake schedules, *Sleep Res.* **13**, 220.

Foret, J. and Lantin, G. (1972). The sleep of traindrivers: An example of the effects of irregular work schedules on sleep, in: *Aspects of Human Efficiency*, ed. W.P. Colquhoun, (English Univ. Press, London), 273–282.

Fuller, C.A., Lydic, R., Sulzman, F.M., Albers, H.E., Tepper, B., and Moore-Ede, M.C. (1981). Circadian rhythm of body temperature persists after suprachiasmatic lesions in the squirrel monkey, *Am. J. Physiol.* **241**, R385-R391.

Gagnon, P. and DeKoninck, J. (1981). Reappearance of EEG slow waves in extended sleep, *Sleep Res.* **10**, 137.

Gagnon, P. and DeKoninck, J. (1982). Reappearance of EEG slow waves in extended sleep with delayed bed-time, *Sleep Res.* **11**, 101.

Gander, P.H., Kronauer, R.E., Czeisler, C.A., and Moore-Ede, M.C. (1984a). Simulating the action of zeitgebers on a coupled two-oscillator model of the human circadian system, *Am. J. Physiol.* **247**, R418–R426.

Gander, P.H., Kronauer, R.E., Czeisler, C.A., and Moore-Ede, M.C. (1984b). Modeling the action of zeitgebers on the human circadian system: Comparisons of simulations and data, *Am. J. Physiol.* **247**, R427–R444.

Gander, P.H., Kronauer, R.E., and Graeber, R.C. (1985). Phase shifting two coupled circadian pacemakers: implications for jet lag, *Am. J. Physiol.* **249**, R704–R719.

Gulevich, G., Dement, W., Johnson, L. (1966). Psychiatric and EEG observations on a case of prolonged (264h) wakefulness, *Arch. Gen. Psychiatry* **15**, 29–35.

Halberg, F. (1959). Physiologic 24-hour periodicity in human beings and mice, the lighting regimen and daily routine, in: *Photoperiodism and Related Phenomena in Plants and Animals*, ed. R.B. Withrow, (AAAS, Washington, D.C.), pp. 803–878.

Halberg, F. (1960). Temporal coordination of physiologic function, *Cold Spring Harbor Symp. Quant. Biol.* **25**, 289–310.

Hoppensteadt, F.C. and Keener, J.P. (1982). Phase locking of biological clocks, *J. Math. Biol.* **15**, 339–349.

Johnson, L.C. (1974). The effect of total, partial and stage sleep deprivation on EEG-patterns and performance, in: *Behavior and Brain Electrical Activity*, eds. N. Bruch and H.L. Altschuler, (Plenum Press, New York).

Jouvet, M., Mouret, J., Chouvet, G., and Siffre, M. (1974). Toward a 48-hour day: Experimental bicircadian rhythm in man, in: *The Neurosciences: Third Study Program*, eds. F. Schmidt and F. Worden, (MIT Press, Cambridge, MA), pp. 491–497.

Kawato, M., Fujita, K., Suzuki, R., and Winfree, A.T. (1982). A three-oscillator model of the human circadian system controlling the core temperature rhythm and the sleep-wake cycle, *J. Theor. Biol.* **98**, 369–392.

Kokkoris, C.P., Weitzman, E.D., Pollak, C.P., Spielman, A.J., Czeisler, C.A., and Bradlow, H. (1978). Long-term ambulatory temperature monitoring in a subject with a hyper-nycthemeral sleep-wake cycle disturbance, *Sleep* **1**, 177–190.

Kopell, N. (1986). Toward a theory of modelling central pattern generators, in: *Neural Control of Rhythmic Movements*, eds. A.H. Cohen, S. Grillner, S. Rossignol, (J. Wiley, New York).

Kopell, N. and Ermentrout, G.B. (1986). Symmetry and phase-locking in chains of weakly coupled oscillators, (to appear).

Kripke, D.F. (1983). Phase-advance theories for affective illnesses, in: *Circadian Rhythms in Psychiatry*, eds. T.A. Wehr and F.K. Goodwin, (Boxwood Press, Pacific Grove, California), pp. 41–69.

Kronauer, R.E. (1982). Reply to R.A. Wever, *Am. J. Physiol.* **242**, R22–R24.

Kronauer, R.E. (1983). Special considerations in interpretation of shifted-sleep experiments, in: *Symposia Abstracts*, 4th International Congress of Sleep Research, Bologna, Italy, p. 64.

Kronauer, R.E. (1984). Modeling principles for human circadian rhythms, in: *Mathematical Models of the Circadian Sleep-Wake Cycle*, eds. M.C. Moore-Ede and C.A. Czeisler, (Raven Press, New York), pp. 105–128.

Kronauer, R.E., Czeisler, C.A., Pilato,S.F., Moore-Ede, M.C., and Weitzman, E.D. (1982). Mathematical model of the human circadian system with two interacting oscillators, *Amer. J. Physiol.* **242**, R3–R17.

Kronauer, R.E., Czeisler, C.A., Pilato, S.F., Moore-Ede, M.C., and Weitzman, E.D. (1983). Mathematical representation of the human circadian system: Two interacting oscillators which affect sleep, in: *Sleep Disorders: Basic and Clinical Research*, eds. M.H. Chase and E.D. Weitzman, (Spectrum, New York), pp. 173–194.

Kronauer, R.E. and Gander, P.H. (1984). Commentary on the article of Daan *et al.*, *Am. J. Physiol.* **246**, R178–R182.

Kronauer, R.E., Strogatz, S.H., and Czeisler, C.A. (1985). Circadian sleep onset rhythm is bimodal across subjects and can be multimodal in individuals, *Sleep Res.* **14**, 300.

Lavie, P. and Scherson, A. (1981). Ultrashort sleep-waking schedule. I. Evidence of ultradian rhythmicity in "sleepability", *Electroencephalogr. Clin. Neurophysiol.* **52**, 163–174.

Lavie, P. and Zomer, J. (1984). Ultrashort sleep-waking schedule. II. Relationship between ultradian rhythms in sleepability and the REM-NONREM cycles and effects of the circadian phase, *Electroencephalogr. Clin. Neurophysiol.* **57**, 35–42.

Lavie, P., Wollman, M., Peled, R., and Zomer, J. (1985). A case study of a hypernycthemeral sleep-wake cycle, *Sleep Res.* **14**, 184.

Lewy, A.J. (1983). Effects of light on melatonin secretion and the circadian system of man, in: *Circadian Rhythms in Psychiatry*, eds. T.A. Wehr and F.K. Goodwin, (Boxwood Press, Pacific Grove, California), pp. 203–219.

Lewy, A.J. and Newsome, D.A. (1983). Different types of melatonin circadian secretory rhythms in some blind subjects, *J. Clin. Endocrinol. Metab.* **56**, 1103–1107.

McCarley, R.W. and Hobson, J.A. (1975). Neuronal excitability modulation over the sleep cycle: A structural and mathematical model, *Science* **189**, 58–60.

McCarley, R.W. and Massaquoi, S.G. (1983). Sleep control mechanisms: A limit cycle model and application to human sleep, *Sleep Res.* **12**, 369.

Miles, L.E.M., Raynal, D.M., and Wilson, M.A. (1977). Blind man living in normal society has circadian rhythms of 24.9 hours, *Science* **198**, 421–423.

Mills, J.N., Minors, D.S., Waterhouse, J.M. (1974). The circadian rhythms of human subjects without timepieces or indication of the alternation of day and night, *J. Physiology*

(London) **240**, 567–594.

Mills, J.N., Minors, D.S., and Waterhouse, J.M. (1978). Adaptation to abrupt time shifts of the oscillator(s) controlling human circadian rhythms, *J. Physiol.* (London) **285**, 455–470.

Minorsky, N. (1962). *Nonlinear Oscillations.* (D. Van Nostrand Company, Inc., Princeton, NJ).

Mistlberger, R., Bergmann, B., and Rechtschaffen, A. (1984). Relationships between adjacent wake and sleep episodes and NREM delta in suprachiasmatic nuclei lesioned rats, *Sleep Res.* **13**, 21.

Moore-Ede, M.C., Sulzman, F.M., and Fuller, C.A. (1982). *The Clocks That Time Us,* (Harvard University Press, Cambridge, MA).

Moore-Ede, M.C., Czeisler, C.A., and Richardson, G.S. (1983). Circadian timekeeping in health and disease, *New England Journal of Medicine* **309**, 469–476 and 530–536.

Moore-Ede, M.C. and Czeisler, C.A. (eds.) (1984). *Mathematical Models of the Circadian Sleep-Wake Cycle*, (Raven Press, New York).

Moore-Ede, M.C., Klerman, E.B., and T.A. Houpt (1986). Mathematical simulation of the effects of rotation shiftwork schedules on circadian sleep-wake cycles and alertness rhythms, *Sleep Res.* **15**, in press.

Moses, J.M., Hord, D.J., Lubin, A., Johnson, L.C., and Naitoh, P. (1975). Dynamics of nap sleep during a 40-hour period, *Electroencephalogr. Clin. Neurophysiol.* **39**, 627–633.

Mrosovky, N. (1986). Sleep researchers caught napping, *Nature* **319**, 536–537.

Nicholson, A., Spencer, M.B., Stone, B., Roehrs, T., and Roth, T. (1984). Sustained performance with short evening and morning sleeps, *Sleep Res.* **13**, 95.

Ohta, T., Ohara, K., Endo, S., Yamamoto, T., Kobayashi, T., and Fukuda, H. (1983). Sleep-wake rhythm and sleep architecture of normal subjects under the entrained, absolute bed-rest condition, *Sleep Res.* **12**, 170.

Pavlidis, T. (1973). *Biological Oscillators: Their Mathematical Analysis*, (Academic Press, New York).

Pittendrigh, C.S. (1981). Circadian systems: Entrainment, in: *Handbook of Behavioral Neurobiology*, vol. 4. *Biological Rhythms*, ed. J. Aschoff, (Plenum Press, New York), pp. 95–124.

Pittendrigh, C.S. and Daan, S. (1976). A functional analysis of circadian pacemakers in nocturnal rodents. I. The stability and lability of spontaneous frequency, *J. Comp. Physiol.* **106**, 223–252.

Richardson, G.S., Carskadon, M.A., Orav, E.J., and Dement, W.C. (1982). Circadian variation of sleep tendency in elderly and young adult subjects, *Sleep* **5**, S82–S94.

Siffre, M. (1964). *Beyond Time*, ed. and transl. H. Briffault, (McGraw-Hill, New York).

Siffre, M. (1972). *Expériences Hors du Temps*, (Fayard, Paris).

Siffre, M. (1975). Six months alone in a cave, *National Geographic* **147** (3), 426–435.

Siffre, M., Reinberg, A., Halberg, F., Ghata, J., Perdriel, G., Slind, R. (1966). L'isolement souterain prolongé. Etude de deux sujet adultes sains avant, pendant et après cet isolement, *Presse Méd.* **74**, 915–919.

Stoker, J.J. (1950). *Nonlinear Vibrations*, (Interscience Publishers, New York).

Strogatz, S.H. and Kronauer, R.E. (1985). Circadian wake-maintenance zones and insomnia in man, *Sleep Res.* **14**, 219.

Strogatz, S.H., Kronauer, R.E., and Czeisler, C.A. (1986). Circadian regulation dominates homeostatic control of sleep length and prior wake length in humans, *Sleep*, in press.

Webb, W.B. (1978a). Sleep and naps, *Spec. Sci. Tech.* **1**, 313–318.

Webb, W.B. (1978b). The forty-eight hour day, *Sleep* **1**, 191–197.

Webb, W.B. and Agnew, H.W., Jr. (1974). Sleep and waking in a time-free environment, *Aerospace Med.* **45**, 617–622.

Webb, W.B. and Agnew, H.W., Jr. (1975). Sleep efficiency for sleep-wake cycles of varied length, *Psychophysiology* **12**, 637–641.

Webb, W.B. and Friedmann, J. (1969). Length of sleep and length of waking interrelations in the rat, *Psychonomic Science* **17** (1), 14–15.

Weber, A.L., Cary, M.S., Connor, N., and Keyes, P. (1980). Human non-24-hour sleep-wake cycle in an everyday environment, *Sleep* **2**, 347–354.

Wehr, T.A. and Goodwin, F.K. (eds.) (1983). *Circadian Rhythms in Psychiatry*, (Boxwood Press, Pacific Grove, California).

Weitzman, E.D., Nogeire, C., Perlow, M., Fukushima, D., Sassin, J., McGregor, P., Gallagher, T.F., and Hellman, L. (1974). Effects of a prolonged 3-hour sleep-wake cycle on sleep stages, plasma cortisol, growth hormone, and body temperature in man, *J. Clin. Endocrinol. Metab.* **38**, 1018–1030.

Weitzman, E.D., Czeisler, C.A., and Moore-Ede, M.C. (1979). Sleep-wake, neuroendocrine and body temperature circadian rhythms under entrainment and non-entrained (free-running) conditions in man, in: *Biological Rhythms and their Central Mechanism*, eds. M. Suda, O. Hayashi, H. Nakagawa, (Elsevier, Amsterdam), pp. 199–227.

Weitzman, E.D., Kronauer, R., Fookson, J., Moline, M., Zimmerman, J., and Ronda, J. (1982). Endogenous oscillators control nap and sleep during non-entrainment, *Sleep Res.* **11**, 221.

Wever, R. (1975). The circadian multi-oscillator system of man, *Int. J. Chronobiol.* **3**, 19–55.

Wever, R. (1979). *The Circadian System of Man*, (Springer-Verlag, Berlin).

Wever, R.A. (1982a). Behavioral aspects of circadian rhythmicity, in: *Rhythmic Aspects of Behavior*, eds. F.M. Brown and R.C. Graeber, (Lawrence Erlbaum Associates, Hillsdale,

NJ), pp. 105–171.

Wever, R.A. (1982b). Commentary on the mathematical model of the human circadian system by Kronauer *et al.*, *Am. J. Physiol.* **242**, R17–R21.

Wever, R.A. (1984a). Properties of human sleep-wake cycles: Parameters of internally synchronized free-running rhythms, *Sleep* **7** (1), 27–51.

Wever, R.A. (1984b). Toward a mathematical model of circadian rhythmicity, in: *Mathematical Models of the Circadian Sleep-Wake Cycle*, eds. M.C. Moore-Ede and C.A. Czeisler, (Raven Press, New York), pp. 17–79.

Winfree, A.T. (1980). *The Geometry of Biological Time*, (Springer-Verlag, Berlin).

Winfree, A.T. (1982a). Human body clocks and the timing of sleep, *Nature* **297**, 23–27.

Winfree, A.T. (1982b). The tides of human consciousness: Descriptions and questions, *Am. J. Physiol.* **242**, R163–R166.

Winfree, A.T. (1982c). Circadian timing of sleepiness in man and woman, *Am. J. Physiol.* **243**, R193–204.

Winfree, A.T. (1983). Impact of a circadian clock on the timing of human sleep, *Am. J. Physiol.* **245**, R497–R504.

Winfree, A.T. (1984). Exploratory data analysis: Published records of uncued human sleep-wake cycles, in: *Mathematical Models of the Circadian Sleep-Wake Cycle*, eds. M.C. Moore-Ede and C.A. Czeisler, (Raven Press, New York), pp. 187–200.

Wollman, M. and Lavie, P. (1986). A hypernycthemeral sleep-wake cycle: Some hidden regularities, Preprint.

Zeeman, E.C. (1977). *Catastrophe Theory*, (Addison-Wesley, Reading, Mass.).

Zulley, J. (1983). Regularity in circadian sleep-wake cycles, *Sleep Res.* **12**, 377.

Zulley, J. (1985). Die circadiane Steuerung des Schlafes, in: *Klinische Psychologie. Psychophysiologische Merkmale klinischer Symptome. Band II. Depression und Schizophrenie*, eds. R. Ferstl, E.R. Rey, D. Vaitl, (Beltz Verlag, Weinheim, FRG), pp. 18–29.

Zulley, J., Wever, R., and Aschoff, J. (1981). The dependence of onset and duration of sleep on the circadian rhythm of rectal temperature, *Pflügers Arch.* **391**, 314–318.

Zulley, J. and Wever, R. (1982). Interaction between the sleep-wake cycle and the rhythm of rectal temperature, in: *Vertebrate Circadian Systems: Structure and Physiology*, eds. J. Aschoff, S. Daan, G. Groos, (Springer-Verlag, Berlin-Heidelberg), pp. 253–261.

Zulley, J. and Campbell, S.S. (1985). Napping behavior during "spontaneous internal desynchronization": Sleep remains in synchrony with body temperature, *Human Neurobiol.* **4**, 123–126.

Index of Authors

Cohen *et al.* (1982), 157.

Colquhoun (1971), 137.

Colquhoun (1972), 82.

Czeisler (1978), 1, 3, 7, 9, 11, 18, 27, 28, 36, 38, 40, 58, 71, 73, 93, 104-106, 109-110, 158, 162.

Czeisler *et al.* (1980a), 10, 18, 40, 58, 62, 71, 73, 77, 79-80, 82, 137, 201.

Czeisler *et al.* (1980b), 40, 62, 82, 93.

Czeisler *et al.* (1981), 10, 102.

Czeisler *et al.* (1982), 10.

Czeisler *et al.* (1985), 24, 90, 92, 97, 102, 209.

Czeisler *et al.* (1986), 24, 82, 90, 92, 97-98, 134, 186, 209.

Daan and Berde (1978), 144-146, 158.

Daan and Beersma (1984), 134-135, 141, 177, 207.

Daan *et al.* (1984), 3, 34, 66, 73, 113, 133-135, 137, 141-144, 148, 150, 177-207, 209.

Dirlich (1984), 144, 146.

Eastman (1984), 47, 113, 118, 134, 144-146.

Elliott *et al.* (1971), 97.

Enright (1980), 144, 146.

Enright (1984), 118, 146.

Ermentrout and Kopell (1984), 157.

Ermentrout and Rinzel (1984), 157.

Fookson *et al.* (1984), 100.

Foret and Lantin (1972), 73.

Fuller *et al.* (1981), 133.

Gagnon and DeKoninck (1981), 137.

Gagnon and DeKoninck (1982), 137.

Gander *et al.* (1984a), 129, 132-133, 144, 207, 210.

INDEX

Journal of
Mathematical Biology

ISSN 0303-6812   Title No. 285

Editorial Board: K. P. Hadeler, Tübingen;
S. A. Levin, Ithaca (Managing Editors); H. T. Banks,
Providence; J. D. Cowan, Chicago; J. Gani, Santa
Barbara; F. C. Hoppensteadt, Salt Lake City;
D. Ludwig, Vancouver; J. D. Murray, Oxford;
T. Nagylaki, Chicago; L. A. Segel, Rehovot

For mathematicians and biologists working in a
wide spectrum of fields, the **Journal of Mathematical Biology** publishes:

- papers in which mathematics is used for a better
  understanding of biological phenomena
- mathematical papers inspired by biological
  research, and
- papers which yield new experimental data
  bearing on mathematical models.

Contributions also discuss related areas of medicine, chemistry, and physics.

Fields of interest: Mathematics, genetics, demography, ecology, neurobiology, epidemiology,
morphogenesis, cell biology, and other branches of
biology.

Abstracted/Indexed in: Biosis, Current Contents,
Excerpta Medica, Inspec, Math. Reviews, Medlars,
Physics Briefs, SCI Abstracts, Technical Information Center/Energinfo, Zentralblatt für Mathematik.

Springer-Verlag
Berlin Heidelberg New York
London Paris Tokyo

For subscription information and sample copies,
contact Springer-Verlag, Dept. ZSW, Heidelberger
Platz 3, D-1000 Berlin 33, W. Germany

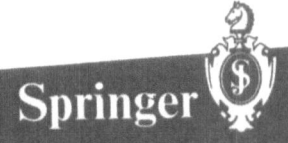

Springer

Volume 17

Mathematical Ecology

An Introduction

Editors: Th.G.Hallam, S.A.Levin

1986. Approx. 87 figures. Approx. 495 pages
ISBN 3-540-13631-2

Contents: Introduction. – Physiological and Behavioral Ecology. – Population Ecology. – Communities and Ecosystems. – Applied Mathematical Ecology. – Subject Index.

Volume 16

Complexity, Language, and Life: Mathematical Approaches

Editors: J.L.Casti, A.Karlqvist

1986. XIII, 281 pages. ISBN 3-540-16180-5

Contents: Allowing, forbidding, but nor requiring: a mathematic for human world. – A theory of stars in complex systems. – Pictures as complex systems. – A survey of replicator equations. – Darwinian evolution in ecosystems: a survey of some ideas and difficulties together with some possible solutions. – On system complexity: identification, measurement, and management. – On information and complexity. – Organs and tools; a common theory of morphogenesis. – The language of life. – Universal principles of measurement and language functions in evolving systems.

Volume 15
D.L.DeAngelis, W.Post, C.C.Travis

Positive Feedback in Natural Systems

1986. 90 figures. Approx. 305 pages. ISBN 3-540-15942-8

Contents: Introduction. – The Mathematics of Positive Feedback. – Physical Systems. – Evolutionary Processes. – Organisms Physiology and Behavior. – Resource Utilization by Organisms. – Social Behavior. – Mutualistic and Competitive Systems. – Age-Structured Populations. – Spatially Heterogeneous Systems: Islands and Patchy Regions. – Spatially Heterogeneous Ecosystems; Pattern Formation. – Disease and Pest Outbreaks. – The Ecosystem and Succession. – References. – Appendices A to H.

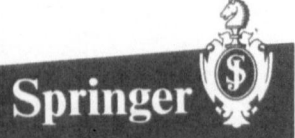

Lecture Notes in Biomathematics